OXFORD MEDICAL PUBLICATIONS

Geriatric problems in general practice

OXFORD GENERAL PRACTICE SERIES

3. Preventive medicine in general practice
   edited by J. A. M. Gray and G. H. Fowler
5. Locomotor disability in general practice
   edited by M. I. V. Jayson and R. Million
6. The consultation: an approach to learning and teaching
   D. Pendleton, P. Tate, P. Havelock, and T. Schofield
8. Management in general practice
   P. M. M. Pritchard, K. B. Low, and M. Whalen
9. Modern obstetrics in general practice
   edited by G. N. Marsh
10. Terminal care at home
    edited by R. Spilling
11. Rheumatology for general practitioners
    H. L. F. Currey and S. Hull
12. Women's problems in general practice
    (Second edition)
    edited by Ann McPherson
13. Paediatric problems in general practice
    (Second edition)
    M. Modell and R. H. Boyd
14. Epidemiology in general practice
    edited by D. Morrell
15. Psychological problems in general practice
    A. C. Markus, C. Murray Parkes, P. Tomson, and M. Johnston
16. Research methods for general practitioners
    David Armstrong, Michael Calnan, and John Grace
17. Family problems
    Peter R. Williams
18. Health care for Asians
    B. R. McAvoy
19. Continuing care: the management of chronic disease
    (Second edition)
    edited by J. C. Hasler and T. P. C. Schofield
20. Geriatric problems in general practice
    (Second edition)
    G. K. Wilcock, J. A. M. Gray, and J. M. Longmore

Geriatric problems in general practice

SECOND EDITION

Oxford General Practice Series 20

G. K. WILCOCK
Professor in Care of the Elderly,
Frenchay Hospital,
University of Bristol; and
Honorary Consultant Physician,
Frenchay Health Authority

J. A. M. GRAY
Community Physician,
Oxfordshire Area Health Authority

J. M. LONGMORE
Principal in General Practice,
Ferring, West Sussex

OXFORD NEW YORK TOKYO
OXFORD UNIVERSITY PRESS
1991

Oxford University Press, Walton Street, Oxford OX2 6DP
Orders by telephone: 0865 242913

Oxford New York Toronto
Delhi Bombay Calcutta Madras Karachi
Petaling Jaya Singapore Hong Kong Tokyo
Nairobi Dar es Salaam Cape Town
Melbourne Auckland

and associated companies in
Berlin Ibadan

Oxford is a trade mark of Oxford University Press

Published in the United States
by Oxford University Press, New York

First published 1982
Second edition 1991

A cataloguing record for this book is available from the British Library

Library of Congress Cataloging in Publication Data
Wilcock, G. K. (Gordon K.)
Geriatric problems in general practice/G. K. Wilcock, J. A. M.
Gray, J. M. Longmore.—2nd ed.
(Oxford general practice series; 20) Oxford
medical publications
Includes bibliographical references and index.
1. Geriatrics. I. Gray, J. A. Muir (John Armstrong Muir)
II. Longmore, J. M. (J. Murray) III. Title. IV. Series.
V. Series: Oxford general practice series; no. 20.
[DNLM: 1. Family Practice. 2. Geriatrics. W1 OX55 no. 20/WT
100 W667ga]
RC952.W45 1991   618.97—dc20   91-1959
ISBN 0-19-261790-7

Typeset by Joshua Associates Ltd, Oxford
Printed in Great Britain by Dotesios Ltd, Trowbridge, Wilts.

Preface to the second edition

Textbooks of geriatric medicine are not prone to set the world alight, nor, at first glance, are they likely to quicken the pulse of prospective readers—for who needs a book on geriatric problems in general practice? Most of us practise geriatric medicine quite well, never having read a textbook on geriatric care in our lives: but when, for whatever reason, we decide to patrol the perimeter of our circle of understanding and see what might lie beyond, we need to start somewhere. We do not at this point immediately claim that our book is the best place to start. Instead of perusing this volume with your mind blank like John Locke's *tabula rasa*, set it aside, and write down on the back of an envelope your chief objectives in caring for your elderly patients— and the main obstacles to achieving these ends. If you find yourself getting into deep water we hope that the pages which follow will be of assistance; alternatively, if the above exercise seems all plain sailing then we aim to show that the ebbing and flowing of geriatric medicine will reveal and hide the odd hostile rock or whirlpool in even our most placid and well-directed consulting rooms.

The main problem, on busy days at least, is that geriatric medicine is so irritating—to the novice, when he or she cannot even start a dialogue with the patient on how to tackle some intractable problem, without first syringing the wax out of his ears, finding a new battery for his hearing aid, and then rummaging through pockets to find reading spectacles—which all takes so long that the patient needs to go to the toilet yet again, but, on his way, as he starts to struggle with his arthritis and a zimmer frame which is two inches too high for him, sheepishly admits that he has left his list of ailments in the car. Do not think that this man must simultaneously have a new zimmer frame, a cataract removed, a prostatectomy, and a new hip. He may need all these things in time, but he may also need a piece of *you*, your sympathy and your advice far more urgently; and you will never find out until you read that list, and your counsel is likely to be entirely wasted if you do not fix that hearing aid—and in so doing you may well have solved what to the patient is his most pressing problem.

We hope that this book will enable the reader to enjoy the challenge of working with old people. This is important because in geriatric medicine are concentrated to an unprecedented degree all the ugly dilemmas of late twentieth-century medicine: the limits and growing side-effects of technology, unlimited demand coupled with finite resources, the ethical questions, the communication gap, the ambivalence towards death, and above all the changing nature of the doctor–patient relationship.

In facing these issues we will be shaping a new and perhaps less stark view of medicine for the years ahead, and we take this opportunity to tip our caps to the historians of the future who may detect in the muddles, insights, and contradictions of geriatric medicine in general practice, the anvil on which was forged one of the brightest parts of twenty-first-century medicine.

J. M. L.

Ferring G. K. W.

June 1991 J. A. M. G.

Preface to the first edition

Most people who work with older patients are caught in a paradox. On the one hand they argue that older people are not qualitatively different from younger people and require a similar approach: the same quality of service, the same respect, the same honesty, and same standard of clinical practice. On the other hand they argue that people *are* significantly different and that their needs are such that they should be given priority for resources, and that doctors and other professionals require special training for their care. In part this paradox can be explained by the fact that most of those who are particularly interested in the problems of older people feel that it is necessary to emphasize that older people are the same, because so many of those who do not have a special interest appear to assume that they are different from younger people by being unable to change or learn, that they are beyond rehabilitation, 'dementing' and 'senile'. Similarly there is a need to argue the case for more services for older people simply to bring them up to the quality of services for other patient groups.

These points only partly explain the paradox. The principal explanation is that the paradox does not really exist at all. Elderly people are the same as younger people; it is elderly *patients* that are different from younger patients. The signs and symptoms of disease, the physical response to disease or trauma or treatment, and the beliefs and attitudes of older patients are slightly, but significantly, different and it is these differences we have tried to summarize in this book.

Furthermore, we have tried to write the book for the doctor seeing, treating, and supporting the elderly person in his own home and that doctor is, of course, the general practitioner. Without junior medical colleagues, pressed for time, without easy access to investigative services, often without the opportunity to undress the patient in warmth and comfort and assailed by the social problems that so often complicate disease in old age the general practitioner has to make the critical decisions. We hope this book will help him to do so.

Our special thanks are due to our families for their support while this book was in preparation, and to Rosemary Lees for her help in producing the book.

Oxford
June 1982

G. K. W.
J. A. M. G.
P. M. M. P.

Acknowledgements

The authors wish to thank Drs M. Suntharalingam and J. Collier for their help in preparing this volume.

Contents

Part I   A philosophy of geriatric medicine in general practice

1 The challenge for general practice

Growth and development are the essence of childhood: but is it correspondingly true that senescence and decay are the essence of old age? In the beginning this may have been true. As nomadic tribes crossed the African plains, they left behind their elders who could not keep up—in specially constructed huts (which have lived on into this century among the Hottentots), where they would await their inevitable demise by lion or jackal. In this world, old age began when you could not keep up. No doubt, and as anthropologists acknowledge, this state of affairs lasted some millennia. Next came the long centuries after the agrarian revolution when to be old was to sit at the hearth stirring a pot and keeping an eye on the grandchildren. Next came the Victorian workhouse, presaging the age of institutionalized care of the elderly. This age held sway until about the time when the first edition of this book was being planned: the early 1980s. Since then an important shift in what it means to be old has begun to take hold, sporadically, and to a varying extent in different parts of the Western World.

In some areas old age (defined as the period of life beyond the retirement age) is turning out to be a period of liberation. Liberation from pointless, or repetitive work, liberation from the ties of dependent children, liberation from the limited horizons that the priorities of the middle years engender, and, most importantly, liberation from financial commitment. Although in the UK there are many, many, poor elderly people, the elderly as a group have never been so rich, and they have never been so well travelled, nor so well informed by the media (most elderly people have at least one television; and magazines designed for the elderly now have six-figure print runs per edition). In the UK, the over-55s account for 25 per cent of the population—but they account for 40 per cent of the nation's net wealth (i.e. the combined wealth of this group is £294 billion, *of which £108 billion is disposable*). People are retiring earlier, and more than half of these elderly people are members of private or company pension schemes, receiving an average of two-thirds of their final salaries. This money is disposable if, as is increasingly the case, it is not necessary to pass on a house to the next generation—who are now likely to be owner occupiers in their own right.

There is no simple equation between money and health, but there is no doubt that the two *are* related. The incidence of almost all diseases, except melanoma and Hodgkin's disease, is positively correlated with poverty and low social class (Whitehead 1987). So it is no surprise to find that the elderly are living longer. There are more of them alive; they have more to live for; they have more to live on—and there is a new confidence in the culture of the elderly. Retirement villages, once only to be found in the USA, are now starting to be built in the UK; travel companies exist specifically to cater for the elderly; and many educational initiatives are largely for the benefit of the elderly. Most significantly, the elderly are doing more for themselves, so ending the cycle of dependency and helplessness. They run their own charities and clubs, they organize their own welfare, they provide their own entertainments and foster their own culture. This trend is only just beginning, and there may well be many readers of this book whose elderly patients are as poor and trapped as ever before (20 per cent of elderly people are totally dependent on State benefits): change does not occur homogeneously, and each individual general practitioner will have their own experience of what old age means in their own localities.

This book is written from the perspective of British general practice—or rather of *one* British general practice. In this practice half the patients are over 65 years old—perhaps the highest proportion in the country, and more than four times the national average. The effect that this has had on our practice has been to prevent us falling into the trap of channelling our natural enthusiasms into the creation of a specialism of Geriatrics in general practice: there are simply too many elderly for them to be hived off as a special group. The care of the elderly is the bulk of our work, and perhaps because of this, our practice offers a glimpse into the future—for the numbers of elderly are rising quite fast, so that many more practices may become like ours. Even if we wanted to, we could not make a specialism out of Geriatrics. We cannot offer special GP-run mini-clinics in the care of the elderly: they would be swamped. We cannot do very comprehensive screening of the elderly: our health visitor has more pressing tasks on her hands. Nor can we hope to offer a fully comprehensive service in the tradition of problem-orientated geriatrics: if we spent time producing a perfect and exhaustive problem list we would have used up all the time allotted for contributing to solving those rather few problems where our intervention might really benefit the patient. So what *can* we do? Are we totally swamped and demoralized by the burden of the elderly? Are we totally constrained to run a reactive service, which simply responds to crises as they occur? Not at all. Strategic planning *is* in evidence, and this is what our book is all about.

We use the word 'challenge' in the title of this chapter rather than some of the more pessimistic terms which have been used to describe the impact of ageing of the population, because we believe that many people have been too pessimistic and that although there is no doubt that the numbers of aged people are going to increase dramatically that does not mean that medical services will not be able to cope. In the last twenty years (1966–86) the proportion of the UK population over the retirement age has risen by 0.5 per cent, from 17.6 per cent to 18.1 per cent—but it is the numbers aged over 75 years which have increased the most: from 5.2 per cent to 6.5 per cent. In absolute figures, this represents a rise in numbers of nearly 700 000

(35 000/year, taking into account the slight increase in the whole UK population). What does a rise of 1.3 per cent in the numbers of people over the age of 75 mean for health care? Their use of hospital beds is tenfold greater than those aged 50–60 years (Fig. 1.1); they are more than ten times as likely to be unable to make a cup of tea for themselves or be able to get to the lavatory (Hunt 1978). In old age, ill health and disability inevitably increase—and it is not a question of doubling; the increase is likely to be by *an order of magnitude*. Fortunately for general practitioners, this large increase is not matched by an order of magnitude increase in consultation

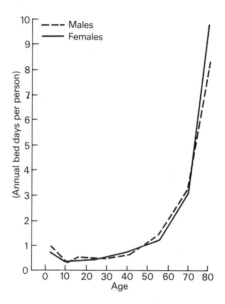

Fig. 1.1. Use of hospital beds (excluding maternity) by patients in different age-groups. From *Population trends* No. 3. HMSO, London (1976).

rates (cf. Fig. 1.6, p. 15). The mean annual GP consultation-rate is 3.5–4.0/ person/year, and this rate only doubles by the age of 80 years. However, because of problems with mobility and social isolation, home visits are often requested by the elderly. Scanning an average morning's visiting list we are not surprised if there is not a date of birth belonging to this century. The challenge for general practice is not to be dumbfounded by this ever-increasing elderly population—but to find ways of enabling one's elderly patients to live the sort of lives they want to live. For most, this will entail living in their own homes until the last possible moment: a good life, followed by a good death—all in the comfort of your own home.

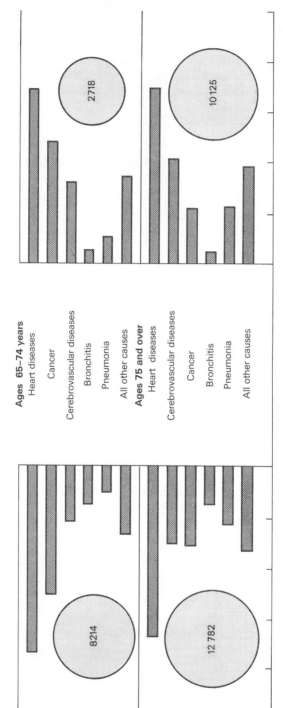

Fig. 1.2. Causes of death in old age. Figures in circles represent the death rates from *all* causes in 1973 per 100 000 population in each age and sex group. (From *Social trends*. HMSO, London (1975).)

Aims and objectives of medicine in old age—background

The common causes of death in old age are shown in Fig. 1.2, although the notorious unreliability of death certificates for old people must be borne in mind when considering these data.

However, the prolongation of life is not one of the principal objectives of medicine in old age; as the motto of the British Geriatrics Society pithily states, the objective is usually to 'Add life to years, not years to life'. Some old people are afraid of death but many are not so much frightened by death as by the prospect of disability, the loss of dignity, and becoming 'a burden' or 'a cabbage'. Indeed some old people look forward to death with pleasure, either because it will relieve them from their present suffering—'I often wish I could just not wake up'—or because they are looking forward to meeting a dead spouse, brothers, or sisters in the life after death.

In spite of the fact that there has been criticism of the medical profession for 'keeping old people alive too long' there is little evidence that this takes place to any significant degree. The expectation of life of old people has not increased dramatically because of the introduction of the National Health Service and it is important to appreciate that there was an increase in the expectation of life before 1948 (Fig. 1.3).

The increase, although small, has been significant for general practitioners because of the high incidence and prevalence of disabling disease. However, the increase in the number of elderly people need not be accompanied by an increase in the numbers of disabled people. Much of disability is caused by disease and unfitness, and one authority has pointed out that even though medicine cannot influence the age of mortality significantly it can postpone the age of onset of disability so that the period of terminal dependency is

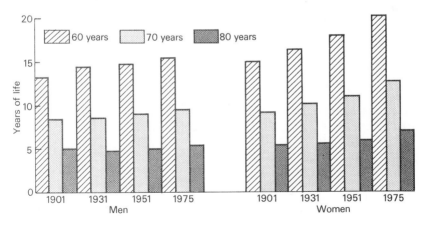

Fig. 1.3. Expectancy of life in Great Britain.

decreased in length, with a fit old age being followed by a short period of dependency before death. The aim of geriatric medicine is therefore to improve the quality of life of older people.

The importance of good health to old people is difficult to overestimate and one sound study (Abrams 1978) of the sources of satisfaction in old age, and the degree to which they were attained, showed clearly how important good health is—second only to 'good neighbours and friends'—and how seldom it is attained (Table 1.1).

In the words of the author of the report, Mark Abrams, 'Clearly, medical care has a very long part to play in determining the quality of life of old people' and he emphasized that health, although second in the list of sources of satisfaction, was lowest in the list when the degree of attainment was assessed.

The main aim of medicine is therefore to improve the quality of life and this aim can be broken down into a number of specific objectives.

- More effective control of disease.
- More effective symptom control.
- The prevention of unfitness.
- The prevention of dependence and handicap.

Table 1.1 How far satisfaction criteria attained:* all aged 65 or more

Potential source of real satisfaction	Proportion naming each source (%)	Degree of attainment				N
		Great extent (%)	Certain extent (%)	Hardly at all (%)	Not at all (%)	
Happy marriage, family	14.1	77	17	2	4 = 100%	232
Helping others	3.7	70	25	4	1	60
Content with lot	11.3	68	28	2	2	186
Sun, warm weather	0.5	67	33	—	—	8
Miscellaneous reason	16.8	66	24	6	4	277
Peace, quiet, solitude	3.8	55	37	4	4	63
Good neighbours and friends	18.4	51	34	12	3	303
Able to get out and about	5.4	48	30	16	6	89
Enough money	9.2	44	37	12	7	151
Good health	14.7	39	46	12	3	242
Total	97.9	Weighted average 58	30	8	4	1611

* In order to obtain a numerically adequate base for each named source of satisfaction this table relates to *all* respondents in the survey.
† Total excludes those who said either that nothing could make for satisfaction in old age, or that they were unable to think of any possible source.
From Abrams, M. (1978). *Beyond three score and ten*, p. 53: Age Concern.

More effective control of disease

This is obviously the foundation of clinical work with older people and is a main theme of this book. However, many diseases are incurable and attention must therefore be paid to the sequelae of disease—symptoms, unfitness, and disability.

More effective symptom control

Many elderly patients are left with distressing symptoms after their disease or diseases have been treated. Some complain about such symptoms; others accept them as inevitable concomitants of 'old age', and specific questions may be necessary to uncover them.

An Age Concern survey of people aged over 75 found only 10 per cent had no physical problem (Table 1.2).

Table 1.2 Proportions suffering from various ailments among people aged 75 or more: England 1977 (expressed as a percentage)

Arthritis, rheumatism	58
Unsteady on feet	49
Forgetfulness	44
Poor eyesight	42
Hard of hearing	36
Backache	36
Breathless after any effort	35
Swelling of feet, legs	33
Giddiness	31
Indigestion, flatulence	29
Always feel tired	29
Heart trouble	21
High blood pressure	21
Headaches	20
Constipation	19
Breathless at night	19
Stomach trouble	18
Long spells of depression	14
Incontinence	11
Toothache, gum trouble	6
Difficulty passing water	5
No. of ailments, average response	5.8
No physical problems	10

From Abrams, M. (1978). *Beyond three score and ten*, p. 55. Age Concern.

In addition to the prescription of appropriate medication or the encouragement of harmless self-medication it is possible to alleviate the effect of many of these symptoms by other means. One way of preventing and alleviating some of these symptoms is to encourage exercise and to try to prevent unfitness.

The prevention of unfitness

There is now good evidence that strength, stamina, skill, and neuromuscular co-ordination can be improved in older people by a programme of fitness training. Furthermore, old people who participate in such programmes report an improvement in morale and feelings of well-being, and these psychological effects may be equally important in the prevention of symptoms such as tiredness and backache.

People who develop a disabling disease are more likely to become unfit than those who do not suffer from chronic disease. There are too few physiotherapists working outside hospital to give such people the type of help they need, and it is often left to the general practitioner to offer advice and encouragement to the disabled old person who would benefit if their fitness were improved.

Prevention of disability and handicap (see p. 169)

These terms are often used as though they were synonymous but it has now been agreed internationally that they should be used to denote different conditions, and this distinction is useful in practice. A *disability* is any restriction or lack of ability to perform an activity in a manner or within the range considered normal for someone of that person's age: for example, the limited hip flexion resulting from osteoarthritis or the limitation in movement and power of the upper limb resulting from the spasticity and contractures on the side of the body affected by a cerebrovascular accident (Wood 1980).

A *handicap* is a disadvantage, such as difficulty with dressing, or preparing food, or reaching the toilet unaided, resulting from a disability. Whether or not a disabled person will be handicapped as a result of her disability is determined not only by the degree of her disability. It is also influenced by her physical environment and by social factors. A person who is so disabled by osteoarthritis of the hips that she cannot climb stairs will be handicapped if she lives in a dwelling in which it is necessary to climb stairs to reach the toilet and bathroom. If that person is rehoused in a dwelling which has no stairs her handicap will be cured even though there has been no change in her degree of disability. The extent to which an individual will be handicapped by her disability is also influenced by the manner in which she has adapted to her disability and by her relationships with other people. With the same degree of disability some people are very much more handicapped than others.

A third term is of particular importance—dependence. A disabled elderly person who lives with relatives, or who has nearby relatives or neighbours who are willing to help her by performing the tasks which she cannot do may not be handicapped, but she will be dependent. Dependence can create problems both for the elderly person and for those on whom she has become dependent.

This distinction between disability and handicap is useful because it allows the contributions by the doctor, physiotherapist, and occupational therapist to be planned in logical sequence. The task of the general practitioner who is faced with a person who is handicapped is to try to minimize the disability by accurate diagnosis, appropriate treatment, and by ensuring that the person complies with treatment. To do this he may have to refer the person to hospital particularly if he is unable to request physiotherapy without hospital assessment. Once doctor and physiotherapist have done as much as they can to reduce the impairment resulting from the disabling disease the occupational therapist can then make her contribution. The objective of occupational therapy is to prevent and cure handicap by helping the disabled person adapt to her environment.

There are two common handicaps in old age—mobility problems and difficulties with self-care.

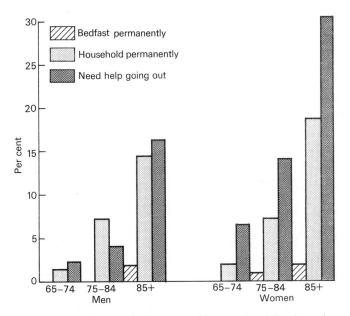

Fig. 1.4. Percentage of men and of women with loss of mobility in each age-group. (From Hunt, A. (1978). *The elderly at home*, p. 69. HMSO, London.)

Mobility problems   Loss of mobility is a central problem in old age which gives rise to many other problems. Mobility problems are more common in women and obviously increase with age (Fig. 1.4).

Audrey Hunt who conducted the survey quoted emphasized the import-ance of immobility by saying that 'one-quarter of those unable to go out, even with assistance, live on their own and are therefore dependent on outsiders for everything that needs to be obtained away from their homes' (Hunt 1978). Furthermore, 42.5 per cent of the bedfast and housebound had not been out of the house for over a year and 18.9 per cent had not been out for over three years.

The causes of these mobility problems were also determined by the survey and what it clearly revealed was that very few people withdraw or 'disengage' from society voluntarily as certain sociologists once argued. Most are immobilized by medical problems (Fig. 1.5).

Self-care problems   The survey revealed that the most difficult self-care tasks were cutting toe-nails and bathing (Table 1.3). In addition the research workers asked about the ability to perform domestic tasks and showed

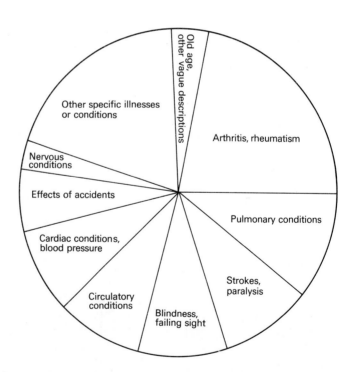

Fig. 1.5.   Causes of being bedfast or housebound. (From Hunt, A. (1978). *The elderly at home*, p. 7. HMSO, London.)

Table 1.3 Percentage in each age-group who are unable to perform each task

	Age-group				
	65–69	70–74	75–79	80–84	85 and over
Elderly persons WEIGHTED	(1409)	(1162)	(679)	(392)	(209)
(unweighted figures)	(725)	(629)	(688)	(375)	(205)
	(%)	(%)	(%)	(%)	(%)
Unable to do without help or totally unable to					
Bath oneself	4.4	11.7	20.2	32.6	51.2
Wash oneself	0.8	1.0	2.3	4.6	7.2
Get to lavatory	0.4	1.3	2.8	5.1	6.2
Get in and out of bed	0.6	1.1	2.7	4.4	4.8
Feed oneself	0.1	0.3	1.3	1.8	2.4
Shave (men), do hair (women)	0.5	0.6	2.5	3.8	4.3
Cut own toe-nails	12.5	21.3	34.6	42.4	56.9
Get up and down steps, stairs	1.6	3.8	10.1	12.8	18.6
Get around house or flat	0.2	0.8	2.2	4.6	6.2
Get out of doors on own	4.4	9.5	16.5	23.5	48.9
Use public transport	5.3	9.3	15.1	23.8	37.9

From Hunt, A. (1978). *The elderly at home*, p. 74. HMSO, London.

difficulties which old people have with house repairs and maintenance, for which there is of course non-statutory help (Table 1.4).

Need and demand

The demands made by old people on general practitioners are heavy but the increase in demand with old age is smaller than would be expected when the increase in morbidity is considered (Fig. 1.6). Demand increases but not, it would appear, in proportion to need. Furthermore there is evidence that the demand is falling (Table 1.5).

Numerous surveys have shown the amount of unreported need among old people at home (Rowntree 1947; Sheldon 1948; Brockington and Lampert 1966). The survey of old people in Edinburgh reported by Profesor Williamson and his colleagues was one of the first careful studies and it revealed that 'men had a mean of 3.26 disabilities of which 1.87 were unknown to the family doctors; women a mean of 3.42 disabilities with 2.03 unknown' (Williamson *et al*. 1964).

Table 1.4 Percentages unable to perform each task (by age)

	Total	Age				
		65–69	70–74	75–79	80–84	85 and over
Elderly persons WEIGHTED	(3869)	(1409)	(1162)	(697)	(392)	(209)
(unweighted figures)	(2622)	(725)	(629)	(688)	(375)	(205)
	(%)	(%)	(%)	(%)	(%)	(%)
Unable to						
Open screw-top bottles*	9.7	5.3	8.4	11.5	18.4	24.4
Do little sewing jobs*	14.9	9.7	11.8	17.1	27.6	35.4
Do jobs involving climbing	43.0	28.0	37.7	57.1	67.3	80.4
Use a frying pan	5.4	2.1	2.8	6.0	13.8	24.9
Make a cup of tea	2.6	0.9	1.4	2.9	6.4	12.9
Cook a main meal	8.8	4.6	6.8	10.0	18.1	26.8
Cut the lawn†	25.8	15.7	20.9	33.4	47.2	56.0
Do heavy jobs in the garden†	47.1	38.4	44.5	55.2	61.0	67.9
Do light jobs in the garden†	19.3	10.0	15.4	27.0	34.7	49.8
Sweep floors	11.3	5.5	8.0	14.8	23.2	34.4
Wash floors	21.7	10.9	15.0	30.8	42.6	62.2
Make fires, carry fuel†	6.0	3.1	4.3	8.6	11.2	17.2
Wash clothes	14.5	6.8	10.8	20.2	29.1	39.7
Clean windows inside	23.6	11.4	17.6	32.3	48.0	65.1
Clean windows outside†	52.5	37.2	50.4	65.0	76.3	84.7
Wash paintwork	23.9	11.6	16.3	32.3	50.5	70.8
Do minor repairs (e.g. fuses)	49.8	35.3	46.0	62.0	73.2	84.2
Repairs and redecoration inside	60.5	11.4	58.3	77.6	87.5	94.4
Repairs and redecoration outside†	49.2	12.0	46.6	53.7	65.6	65.6

* Bedfast informants were asked about these tests. They are assumed to be unable to do the other tests.

† Informants who would not have to perform these tasks (e.g. because they had no garden) are included in the base figures so that the figures given show the percentages of all elderly for whom the tasks present problems. The percentages to whom these do not apply are: lawn 29.7 per cent, garden 22.6 per cent, solid fuel fires 55.8 per cent, windows outside 3.1 per cent, redecoration outside 35.9 per cent.

From Hunt, A. (1978). *The elderly at home*, p. 81. HMSO, London.

The reasons for the low level of demand among elderly people are complex. Some are due to trends in general practice which inhibit demand but the more important factors are the beliefs and attitudes of old people themselves. For this reason we need to consider the ways in which older patients differ from those of working age, physically, socially, and psychologically (see p. 16).

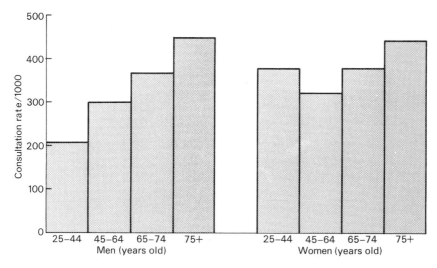

Fig. 1.6. Consultation rates per 1000 population. From *Morbidity statistics from general practice*, Studies on medical and population studies No. 14. HMSO, London.)

Table 1.5 Average percentage in rate between 1971 and 1978 as percentage of 1971 rate—Great Britain

Age-Group	Consultation	Attendances	Visits
45–64	−1.0	+8.6	−38.9
65–74	−17.5	−11.5	−28.5
75 and over	−29.3	−19.8	−34.9

Derived from the general household survey in Billsborough, J. S. (1981). Do patients consult the doctor less often than they used to? *J. R. Coll. Gen. Pract.* 31, 91–105.

2 Setting objectives

The aim of this book is to help general practitioners to improve the quality of care they give to older people. Its specific objectives are:

1. To summarize the physical, social, and psychological differences which distinguish older people from younger people.
2. To emphasize the practical implications of these differences.
3. To summarize the differences in the signs and symptoms of disease in old age and give guidance on the differential diagnosis of common problems such as falling or incontinence.
4. To outline the differences in clinical pharmacology which have to be borne in mind when prescribing for older people and to suggest ways in which compliance can be improved.
5. To review the common clinical conditions encountered in old age, both acute and chronic, and give guidance on management options.
6. To advise the general practitioner on the steps that he or she can take to prevent disease in old age.
7. To provide information on the difficulties that elderly people have with general practice, and to suggest ways by which these may be minimized.
8. To make suggestions to readers about ways in which the primary care team can work more effectively in providing support for elderly people.
9. To suggest ways in which general practitioners can play a part in the local community to improve voluntary and social services for elderly people.
10. To illustrate some of the ethical dilemmas which are likely to confront those who care for the elderly.

In what way does disease differ in old age?

Before answering this question it is essential to emphasize that there is no such thing as 'old age' as a condition different from 'young age'. Old age is a condition like high blood pressure, and there is no sharp cut-off point, even though terms such as hypertension and normotension would seem to indicate that there are two states. The older the age, the more the impact of ageing and the related factors which alter the presentation of disease. Ages such as 65 or 75 as cut-off points for classifying old people are simply arbitrary points chosen by economists or health service planners. This is shown in the graph below.

The second important point to emphasize is that elderly people differ from one another in many more ways than they resemble one another, and the

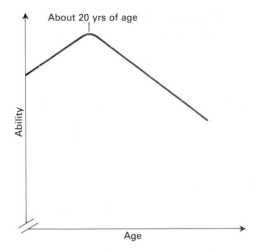

Fig. 2.1. A graph of ability against age.

corollary of this is that older people differ biologically from one another more than younger people. The range of physical and psychological abilities in a group of 80-year-olds, for example, is much greater than the range in a group of 20-year-olds. Therefore all generalizations about older people, including those in this book, must be treated with caution.

Clinical pointer

It is sometimes useful to forget an individual's chronological age and the influence of chronological age on decision making can be reduced by asking yourself: 'What would I do if this person were 35?'

Accepting all these reservations, let us now consider the ways in which disease differs in older age-groups.

1. The sharp distinction between physical and mental health is more often blurred.
2. Medical and social problems are intertwined; all medical problems have social consequences and all social problems should be considered as having medical causes until proven otherwise (pp. 194–7).
3. Presentation of disease is often atypical; classic textbook presentations are less often seen.

4. Elderly people are more susceptible to the side-effects of treatment, so the benefit-to-risk ratio of treatments differs in old age.
5. The beliefs and attitudes of older people are different, and this influences presentation (p. 20).
6. The health problems of older people dominate all health services with the exception of paediatrics and obstetrics. For example, the group in which renal transplantation has been increased more quickly is the over-65s.
7. Good health is more important to older people (in their own estimation) as a contribution to the quality of life than it is to younger people, in part because the younger age-groups are inclined to take good health for granted.

What are the objectives of health care for older people?

It is helpful here to consider the distinction between objectives concerned with *outcome* and those concerned with the *process* of care. The validity of this distinction and the tendency to promote *outcome* over *process* has long been almost universal. The reason for this preference seems to be that *process* can go wrong: all too often it does not lead to the intended *outcome*. For example, a study that shows that a particular drug safely reduces post-operative prothrombin time is a *process* study because it is just one step on the road to reducing post-operative deep venous thrombosis. A DVT is not really an outcome, though, as on its own, it does not matter very much. The argument is: If you prevent DVTs, you will prevent pulmonary embolism. On this view, pulmonary embolism is an end-point—and a study which looks at pulmonary emboli is to be preferred to one that looks only at DVTs. Supposing that the drug *did* produce a marked reduction in the frequency of pulmonary embolism: is this the end of the story? No: if the pulmonary emboli were very small, and hardly clinically noticeable, the benefits of giving the drug would be minimal. So choose another end-point: say, *large* pulmonary emboli.But what if those who got the big pulmonary emboli were, in fact, those destined to die anyway from the procedure? So the real question is (it might be thought): does the drug prevent deaths? Surely death is a valid end-point. The answer has to be no. Perhaps by some pharmacological quirk, the drug only prevents death if the patient is demented, institutionalized, or permanently suicidal. This shows that death is no more valid an end-point than any of the others mentioned (prothrombin time, DVTs, pulmonary emboli, large pulmonary emboli, and even death itself are all *process*)—and what is the process a process towards? The only valid answers are those that are frustratingly vague: such as happiness, quality of life, or freedom. Even freedom is a question of *process* not outcome, because freedom on its own has no value: it has always got to be freedom to do *something*. If the drug in question prolonged the prothrombin time, reduced the frequency of DVTs and large and small pulmonary emboli, increased survival irrespective of whether the patient was demented or suicidal, and increased freedom, must this drug be a good thing, assuming that there are no side-effects? Not necessarily: if the freedom which is increased is the freedom from inhibitions, the drug might have the disastrous consequence that those who have taken it might act out all their agression and become post-operative murderers.

So the distinction between *process* and *outcome* is ultimately unsustainable: if our objectives are measurable, they must be *process—and they are still likely to be process* if they are vague and unmeasurable. Even so, it is worth pointing out that there is a gradation within *process* objectives: i.e., those objectives which we think will count as small steps to achieving larger objectives. What counts as a larger objective? Generally, a larger objective is one that the patient or his carer would embrace. For example, the patient himself is unlikely to worry much about whether his GP has his notes in chronological order (a tertiary objective which leaves the patient cold). But the GP might think that this is important in enabling him to diagnose more quickly and accurately (a secondary objective which the patient might warm towards). Accurate diagnosis is only desirable because it sometimes enables a primary objective to be realized: increased well-being (through specific treatment).

Primary objectives	Secondary objectives	Tertiary objectives
To improve the quality of life	To diagnose accurately	To improve access to services
To improve function	To prognosticate accurately	To communicate with other professionals
To halt decline	To prevent the preventable	To refer cases as needed
To prevent premature death in old age	To anticipate future problems	To know the local health needs
To minimize the impact of health problems	To provide an acceptable environment for the delivery of health care	To measure progress towards meeting primary and secondary objectives
To provide prompt treatment–without side-effect (physical or psychological)	To sympathize with the patient's predicament to augment the patient's will to get better	

The reason for displaying the objectives as above is to emphasize that we should be wary of spending time outside the affairs of the left-hand column, unless we are quite sure that engaging in the right-hand column will yield left-hand column results.

The population of elderly people is constantly changing as people who reach what is socially defined as old age bring to old age a different experience. The term used by epidemiologists is 'cohort'. For example, the cohort of men who fought in and survived the First World War is dying out—and is being replaced by a cohort of men who fought in the Second World War. Cohorts change in three ways.

- Changes in attitude
- Changes in wealth
- Changes in health

Changes in attitude

Many very elderly people have low expectations and a limited sense of their rights. This is scarcely surprising in a generation brought up to know hard times and repeated disappointments.

Case study

Mr. D. is living in a damp council house. Social and health workers have been trying for months to improve his housing and reduce the damp-ness without success. They finally go to see him to tell him that they think it is impossible to solve his problems; but Mr.D. consoles them:

'Never mind, in 1915 I was up to my waist in mud and water, so this is not too bad.'

Checklists of disappointments experienced by elderly people which have taught them not to raise their hopes too high

---

- The 'war to end all wars'
- 'It will be over by Christmas'
- 'Homes fit for heroes'
- 'Peace in our time'

Older people are changing, and those who are now becoming older belong to trade unions or professional associations, and have known more prosperity and expect a better deal from life. The newest cohort to become elderly is part of the consumer generation.

Changes in wealth

These are described on p. 3.

Changes in health

Some diseases are closely related to the ageing process (pp. 55–139) and do not therefore change significantly in prevalence with time. For example, it appears that the prevalence of dementia among people aged 80 is not changing significantly.

Other diseases, however, are caused by environmental factors: either factors in the physical environment, such as air pollution, or in the social environment—which lead to changes in life-style and health habits.

These diseases do change with time and occur with different prevalences in different cohorts.

Some diseases are increasing and some are decreasing.

Brain teaser

List three diseases of old age that are increasing and three diseases of old age that are decreasing.

In general, people now aged 70 are bigger and fitter than the 70-year-olds of the past. There are two reasons for this.

1. People are now arriving at old age fitter and stronger because children have been getting fitter and stronger each generation.
2. Medical treatment such as treatment of cataract or osteoarthritis of the hip or coronary arteriosclerosis is more effective than it was.

The survival curve has therefore changed in shape this century. What will be the impact of these changes in the future?

The optimist's view   The optimists believe that the effect of these trends will be to keep people fitter longer—with the result that they will have a shorter terminal illness, and only a short period of heavy dependency before death. On this view, people will, in the words of Sir Richard Doll, 'die young as late as possible'.

The pessimist's view   The pessimists, however, believe that the increase in life-span which we are observing may be accompanied by a postponement of the age at which heavy dependency occurs, but will also result in an increase in the duration of terminal dependency.

These two positions are set out in Fig. 2.2.

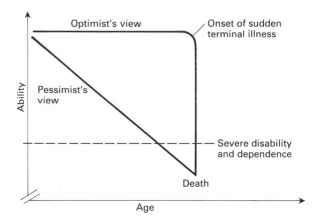

Fig. 2.2.   Two patterns of decline in the last five years of life.

Nobody knows what the effect will be. Undoubtedly as a result of the changes that have taken place which have resulted in an increase in life-span and health, some people will survive fit and active until a short terminal illness occurs—whereas others who would have previously died will survive with a much longer period of heavy terminal dependency. It is the mix of these different types of life pattern which will determine the overall health pattern—but we do not have sufficient information to allow us to say what the final outcome will be.

3 Thinking about the problem of old age

The objective of this chapter is to describe the nature of the health problems that occur in old age. These health problems can be considered in two ways: either classifying them by presentation or by cause.

Classification by presentation
1 Declining physical ability
2 Declining psychological ability
3 Impaired quality of life
4 Life-threatening conditions
5 Conditions which impose strain on informal supporters

Classification by cause
1 Ageing
2 Disease
3 Loss of fitness
4 Social problems and pressures

Common presentations of disease in old age

Declining physical capacity

Physical capacity increases for about two decades after birth and then, following the turning point, there is a decline in physical capacity (Fig. 3.1). Ageing becomes a dominant process when the phase of growth and development comes to an end and ageing leads inevitably to a certain loss of functional ability. However, the time at which capacity starts to decline and the rate of decline are, in almost everyone, determined not solely by ageing but by ageing and loss of fitness.

The impact of loss of fitness is evident in Fig. 3.2. Imagine that X is the capacity level to walk 400 yards and climb a flight of stairs. For the individual who has an upstairs toilet and lives 400 yards from the post office and shops, this capacity therefore marks the threshold of dependency. Observe the rate of decline for Mr A and Mr B. Mr A has kept himself reasonably but not obsessively fit, cycling to the shops at the weekend instead of driving. Mr B on the other hand has not kept himself so fit. Mr A drops below the dependency threshold at age x, and Mr B at age y. Therefore small differences in the rate of dependency at which individuals lose fitness can have a major impact on the age at which they become dependent.

Now let us consider the impact of disease. When disease develops there is obviously an acceleration in the best possible rate of decline, as shown in Fig. 3.2.

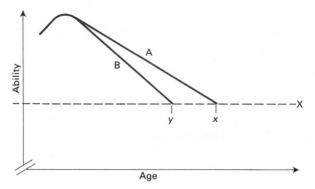

Fig. 3.1.   A graph of physical capacity against age in two individuals.

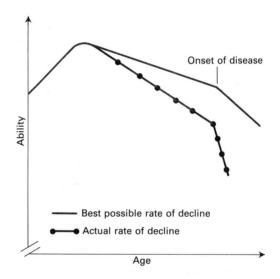

Fig. 3.2.   The impact of disease on the rate of decline of physical capacity.

However, even more serious is the fact that people who develop disabling diseases often lose fitness even more quickly than elderly people of the same age who do not have a disabling disease. Thus the fitness gap grows wider faster. There are two reasons for this which will be discussed in the next section of the chapter.

The final point to make about the decline in physical capacity that takes place with age is that research has shown that this decline can be reversed at any age either by treatment of disease or by helping individuals regain fitness.

Declining intellectual ability

If intellectual ability is plotted against time the same shape of graph is obtained as was seen for physical ability.

Although the research on changing psychological abilities is less than the research on changing physical ability, it is probable that there is a gap between the best possible rate of decline and the actual rate of decline. The reason for this gap is principally due to lack of stimulation and this is a particular problem for people suffering from sensory deprivation due to visual or hearing impairment and isolation. The research done on the effect of isolation and sensory deprivation using brainwashing techniques demonstrates that very severe effects can be produced quickly in young fit people and on the basis of this it is reasonable to suppose that sensory deprivation and isolation in old age also leads to a number of intellectual changes and emotional disorders.

In addition there may be a certain type of loss of intellectual 'fitness' resulting from the fact that younger people may not correct and argue with very elderly people in the same way that they would with their peers. It often seems kinder to let mistakes pass when dealing with very elderly people but it is the correcting of mistakes by other people which helps us keep well-orientated.

Many diseases cause an acceleration in the rate of decline in intellectual ability. This may occur over a short period of time, for example as a result of acute infection, or over a long period of time as a result of the development of Alzheimer's disease or one of the other less common causes of dementia.

As with the onset of physical disease, the gap between the best possible and actual levels of intellectual ability probably widens more quickly after the onset of Alzheimer's disease because the person with Alzheimer's disease is more likely to be isolated, is unlikely to have sensory deprivation countered, and may be treated differently solely on account of her Alzheimer's disease.

Case of the labelled clock-watcher

Mrs S was 81 and had early-stage Alzheimer's disease for which she had been referred for assessment to the Geriatric Unit. She was observed one morning going to the shops at 7.00 by the warden of her sheltered flat. The warden kindly rushed out and brought her home but five minutes later she was off down the road again and was brought home under protest, and as her distress showed no signs of abating the general practitioner was called, who administered a tranquillizer which caused her to sleep all day. She turned up for a 7.30 p.m. bingo session at 5.25, was led back to her flat, came down again, was taken back to her flat. The warden phoned for the GP again, the neighbour phoned for the son, and Mrs S was extremely distressed, saying that people were trying to kill her.

It was then discovered that her son, instead of turning the clock back an hour the previous evening, the autumn equinox, had turned it forward, but no-one thought of finding out what Mrs S had thought the time was. All her behaviour was assumed to be due to her Alzheimer's disease.

Question of competence   As intellectual ability declines, the competence of an individual becomes impaired but whether or not this is a problem depends upon the tasks that they have to carry out, as shown in the diagram. The assessment of competence is not therefore something that can be carried out in isolation but has to be done in the context of the decisions which the old person has to make.

Impaired quality of life

Much of the effort of health services is rightly directed towards improving the functional ability of older people but it is equally important to tackle those problems which impair quality of life.

1 By providing more effective management of disorders which are treatable, if not curable; and there is no doubt that the management of disorders such as depression, incontinence, and visual problems could be improved.
2 By the provision of more effective support for people suffering from incurable or untreatable conditions.

Life-threatening illness

The common causes of death in old age are:

Heart diseases
Cancer
Cerebrovascular diseases
Bronchitis
Pneumonia

The emphasis on medical care in old age is to provide services which will reduce disability, improve the quality of life, and lessen the burden on carers, but elderly people should not be excluded from potentially life-saving treatments solely because of their age.

Obviously the choice of individuals for treatment is one which has many serious ethical implications. This will be discussed in the section on terminal care.

Providing support for relatives

The most common type of care in old age is self-care; the second most important type of care is informal care provided by friends, neighbours, and, most frequently, the family. When elderly people are involved in informal

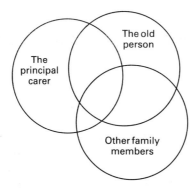

Fig. 3.3.   Main actors in the drama of informal care of the elderly.

care there are usually three main players in the drama. For each person and their principal carer there is a breaking-point, a point at which the relative says 'I cannot go on.' The level of the breaking-point varies from one family to another, depending partially on the relationship between the old person and the principal carer. Not all old people are nice old people, and those who are not were often not nice young people. This means that they may not have been particularly satisfying as parents, and an interesting analogy is to consider that when children leave home to start their own adult lives they owe their parents something. They are in debt, and the parents are in credit. As the parents grow older, they draw upon their credit, but some old people end up in overdraft—depending on how much credit they had to start off with, and how many times they drew on that credit.

The patterns of family breakdown and the challenges for the general practitioner vary from one instance to another. Sometimes the story is one of gradual decline with a gradual increase in strain.

On other occasions the level of tension in the family increases dramatically even though the old person's condition has not changed.

Mrs M turned up in her GP's surgery one day and said that she 'couldn't go on' and that her mother had to be taken into long-stay care. What emerged over the next week was that the principal problem causing concern to Mrs M was the pending divorce of her daughter. Her daughter lived 200 miles away and was making impractical demands on her mother's time, but the strain was such that Mrs M felt unable to continue caring for her own mother.

The third pattern is the pattern of repeated episodes, with each small crisis raising the level of tension in the family. The family which phones on Friday requesting a home visit because their elderly relative has developed incontinence may accept a visit on Monday—but a weekend dealing with an incontinent old person may permanently and irreversibly raise the level of tension until a very small problem takes the family beyond breaking-point.

4 Some ethical issues in geriatric medicine

It is not our place to prescribe a system of ethics to cover geriatric medicine—but to discuss geriatric medicine *without* reference to any ethical matter would be to miss its kernel. Ethical problems often arise in geriatric medicine when there is a conflict between the four 'universal' principles (Beauchamp and Childress 1983) which are often used to inform and guide moral reasoning in the medical world: respect for autonomy of the patient, and the duties of justice, beneficence, non-maleficence (e.g. *primum non nocere*—first do no harm). When there is a conflict of principles in our own practice of geriatric medicine we tend to give priority to autonomy, and this view may be encapsulated in the principle: If the patient's views are known, comply with them (more-or-less irrespective of the views and interests of other marginally affected parties).

Why does this principle have especial significance in geriatric medicine? The position is not that there are any unique features of geriatric medicine requiring some new form of ethical reasoning. The answer is simply that old people may be free of dependents, whose needs and views need to be taken into account when deciding which ethical principles apply in any given instance. For example, I am called to the bedside of a previously well forty-year-old bread-winner who clearly has deep venous thrombosis in one of his legs. I explain the diagnosis to him. He tells me that he wants to be looked after at home. I know that I cannot offer nearly such good treatment at home—so what should I do?

Simple application of the principle of priority to the patient's wishes indicates that I should buckle down to daily calcium heparin injections at home with whatever haphazard arrangements I can make for warfarin anti-coagulation. But is this fair on his wife and children? I ask them for their opinion and they confirm that they do not want admission to hospital either. After a thorough assessment, my next step is to ensure that their decisions are based on the correct assumptions. I may regard it as my duty to explore why they are against hospital admission. Is their objection a valid one (e.g. that the father detests authority or institutionalization)—or is the reasoning more tenuous (e.g. a fear of hospitals based on a former bad experience in hospital)? If the latter, then it could be regarded as my duty to do my best to disperse the tenuous reasoning, and replace it by something more robst, something more in the public domain of reasoning, rather than private fears and doubts. I am justified, it could be argued, in dispelling these both because of my duty to try to do the best for my patient and from a duty to try to prevent harm to his dependents, should a fatal pulmonary embolism ensue. Some practitioners would go further, and say that it would be correct, if initial attempts fail to change his mind, that I should deliberately overstate the risk of pulmonary embolism in trying to tip the balance in favour of admission to hospital—adding graphic descriptions of a painful death—if all other means of persuasion fail.

But what is the position with an older person with no dependent children who is spending his last years in his beloved bungalow with his aged wife? If he develops a DVT and declines my offer of admission to hospital am I justified in trying to force on him my style of public reasoning (the sort which would stand up in a court of law)? Let us suppose that he does not want to die—and also that he is not afraid of dying—and that his chief fear is of leaving his home. He would like to die at home—when the time comes. In these set of circumstances our principle (*If the patient's views are known, comply with them*) carries even more weight than in our example of a younger man—because there is little point in being an elderly person if you cannot conduct your life according to your own principles (i.e. respect for autonomy assumes maximum importance, as other aims such as general beneficence become less relevant). At this point someone might counter that respect for autonomy is valid for all ages—but it is possible that someone might reasonably forgo autonomy in his or her middle years in order to try to maximize it in his old age, but in old age such putting off is less likely to have beneficial consequences. In our practice we have made this principle of complying with the patient's views the cornerstone of our ethical position *vis-à-vis* our elderly patients because of the above considerations. Recognizing his liberty also confers a dignity on the old person—and this is the main attraction of this philosophy. Another important attraction is that it becomes quite clear to the patient that his doctor is his agent and advocate—and not the embodiment of bureaucratic powers. Sending this clear message to the patient is central to the process of augmenting the patient's trust in his doctor—and as we have illustrated elsewhere, where there is no trust, there can be little healing.

It is important to point out that this sort of thinking only makes sense if a thorough geriatric assessment has taken place, to ensure that no other simply treatable pathologies exist.

There are also adverse consequences of giving pre-eminence to this principle. (As with drugs, all ethical principles have side-effects.) The most serious is that, on occasion, the principle is self-defeating. In other words, by enabling the patient's present wish to be fulfilled we limit our ability to fulfil all subsequent wishes. For example, a patient who has a small stroke, and declines investigation may go on to have a larger stroke—so severe that he is not able to tell us what he wants, so that we have to act for him and, perhaps, do things to him to which he would not give consent, were he able to express an opinion. This objection is less serious in the elderly patient than it is in a younger patient, who may have to lead a lifetime in the shadow of the consequences of one unfortunate choice. In the elderly, who have already had the bulk of their life, the future might be said to matter less: it is short—and if they are living on borrowed time anyway (having survived a number of usually fatal illnesses), any gain is a boon, and it is worth risking damage to the patient's state of health.

Another problem with our chief principle is that a patient may initially choose not to go to hospital. He may subsequently change his mind, after the initially preventable complications have become irreversible. In these circumstances the patient may blame the doctor, saying 'Why did you not do more to persuade me to go to hospital?' There is no very satisfactory reply to this. Suffice it to say that in our experience it has not happened to any of our patients. If it did, the best thing to do might be to apologize and explain why one did what one did (because of respect for the patient's choices). Sometimes the answer to the question 'What shall I do?' may be as unhelpful as Hamlet's to his mother: 'Good lady . . . not this, by no means, that I bid you.' In this case, perhaps it is right for the doctor to prescribe whatever philosophy he thinks is right.

Is there a way of formalizing our principle of doing only what the patient wants? One possibility is for the patient to arrange for an enduring power of attorney. This is a legal document which gives authority to a named person to act as a proxy in health care matters when the patient is no longer competent to make decisions for him or herself.

Living wills

One new development (which does not require the services of a lawyer) in this regard has been the so-called 'living will', in which the patient specifies the treatment to which he or she will give consent—should certain illnesses arise. For example, a living will might go like this.

Living will: declaration to be signed by the patient

Name: Mr Mrs Miss Ms   Date of birth:
Address:

Next of Kin: Mr Mrs Miss Ms
                     Address

                     Telephone number

If I have a stroke and am unconscious, I hereby decline to give my consent to the passing of a nasogastric or orogastric tube for the purposes of feeding and nourishment—whether or not I am able to swallow. I include in this prohibition any form of artificial feeding. I understand what a stroke is. This has been explained to me by Dr Longmore of 22 Ferring St, Ferring, West Sussex who has been my general practitioner for 4 years. I understand that a stroke entails an injury to my brain which is enduring and leads to loss of function. It can be brought about either by a block in an artery or other blood vessel, or a burst in a blood vessel, or by a fall in my blood pressure which results in part of my brain dying from lack of oxygen. I fully understand that one loss of function may be my ability to swallow. It may be tempting for my doctors (with the best of intentions) to prolong my life by feeding me via a tube passed into the stomach (a nasogastric or orogastric tube). I realize that the outlook after a stroke is variable. Some people who, in the weeks after a stroke, remain unconscious and unable to swallow may recover somewhat. Knowing this does not alter my views on what I want for myself. Tube feeding may prolong the process of dying, and this is why I will not allow it for myself. If I am unconscious after a stroke, please ensure that I am not apparently distressed or restless (sedate me if necessary) and allow nature to take its course. If I remain unconscious after the stroke I do not want antibiotic treatment for pneumonia or any other infection, and I hereby do not consent to this treatment. I allow that for the first few days afer a stroke I may need hydrating with water delivered through a vein in order that my doctors may determine the extent of my stroke, and the likelihood of significant recovery. I reject continuation of such hydration for more than a few days unless my doctors confidently believe they can predict a good likelihood (more than . . . per cent) of a substantial recovery towards an independent, self-directed, self-aware and satisfying life.

If I develop any other similar brain disease or injury which renders me permanently incapable of giving informed consent, I hereby require that the treatments outlined above shall not be given to me.

If I develop an abdominal aortic aneurysm and I am over 80 years old, I hereby expressly refuse consent for surgery should the aneurysm appear to burst or start leaking. I fully appreciate that surgery may be life-saving, but given that I am over 80 years old and have already had a good stretch of life, I do not want to lay myself and my relatives open to the problems arising from unsuccessful surgery. Dr Longmore has explained to me exactly what aneurysm is. It is a ballooning of the main artery in the body. It leaks because the artery's wall has been weakened and torn. I understand that the untreated mortality from this condition is 100 per cent. With surgery, some people (a small minority) survive. I am trying to avoid an unsatisfactory death, either on the operating table, or, after surgery, in an intensive care unit where I will be unconscious and unable to control events.

If I develop respiratory failure as a complication of a lung disease which is permanent and incurable, or if I develop serious pneumonia, such that I am unconscious or nearly so, and am unable to breathe on my own—I hereby specifically withhold my consent to mechanical ventilation. I understand what mechanical ventilation entails. Dr Longmore, of 22 Ferring St, Ferring, West Sussex, who has been my doctor for 4 years, has explained to me the nature and purpose of mechanical ventilation. I fully appreciate that this system of treatment may be life-saving, but given that I am over 80 years old and have already had a good stretch of life I do not want to lay myself and my relatives open to the problem arising from mechanical ventilation.

This will shall lapse if it is not renewed by me within 5 years from the date of its signature.

Signature

Date . . .

Witnesses   (One)   Name:
                                  Address:

                 (Two)   Name:
                                  Address:

Read over by (or to) the above named, and signed by the above named in our presence, and by us in his/her presence.

Signature of witness one   Date

Signature of witness two   Date

Declaration to be signed by the above person's general practitioner.

I have read the above declaration and can confirm that these arrangements are the wishes of my patient, and I further confirm that my patient is of sound mind and fully able to appreciate the meaning of this document. I have taken steps to ensure that the patient has been placed under no undue pressure or coercion to sign this document. I myself have no personal or pecuniary interest in the above patient's death.

Signature

Date

Signed copies of this document are lodged with the next of kin (address as above), and in the patient's records (registration number . . .) at the Surgery, 22 Ferring Street, Ferring, West Sussex, and the records at Southlands Hospital (registration number . . .).

This sort of living will can be adapted in many ways. For example a living will may be drawn up by a patient with advanced cancer in order to limit the use of chemotherapy, or by people who fear they may become demented. Whilst they are still of sound mind they may, for example, decide to indicate that if they become demented and persistently refuse help and admission to hospital or a nursing home, they will agree to a trial period of two weeks in an approved establishment, only to be returned home if they express a wish to do so (so recognizing the fact that many such patients will think that they *are* at home after two weeks in a nursing home or rest home).

The background to these choices is the fact that many elderly patients who are of sound mind are chiefly concerned that they should not be a burden on their relatives. They see life as if it were a baton in a relay race: they have passed it on to their offspring, and the last thing they want is for their worn-out bodies to be a millstone around the necks of those who are still in the running. Other old people, not necessarily more selfish, may choose to have nothing to do with this line of thought. The main thing is for the general practitioner to be aware that patients' views will differ markedly, and so to make sure that all the patients signing living wills understand what the consequences will be.

There are numerous problems with living wills.

- Their legal status is uncertain in the UK (in the USA the Supreme Court has recently upheld their legal validity). The uncertainty exists in the UK because there is no case law referring to them—i.e. no one has contested the validity of a living will in a court of law. If a contest did arise, with the patient charging that battery with substantial damage occurred because his or her living will was knowingly ignored, it might be possible for the doctor to defend himself by reference to a breach of professional ethics. This defence in the UK might be as unsuccessful as similar defences have proved in the USA.

- Problems may arise if the doctor *does* comply with the terms of a living will, acts contrary to normal medical practice, and injury occurs to the patient as a result.

- A living will may not be available when it is needed; for example, the patient may fall ill away from home. One way round this problem is for the patient to wear a 'Medic-Alert' bracelet containing the fact that a living will exists, and where it can be found. Another possibility is to use the 'Smart Card', which is a credit-card sized piece of plastic with a computer-readable text on it. This may be accessed by a reading device held in general practitioner's surgeries and in hospitals. Their use is not widespread at present but this may change.

- If a patient wanting to sign a living will is dreading the thought that in extreme old age he or she will be a burden to relatives, he may word the document to make his reasoning manifest. In one sense this is a wise precaution, because it demonstrates in a very strong way that the patient is in full possession of his faculties—and this is essential to any attempt to try to guarantee the will. However, when the relatives read the will, they may then feel very guilty: it is because of them that the old person is denying himself possibly life-saving (or at least life-prolonging) treatment. This may bring about exactly what the old person fears—either through suppression of the living will or through excessive guilt after its execution. Therefore the general practitioner may feel that it is wise to advise that the wording of the will is in terms of what the patient wants for himself, and for his own benefit.

- Once the patient falls ill, his soundness of mind at the time of writing the living will may be called into question. A simple way to try to avoid this problem is for the general practitioner or his nurse to do a mini-mental-state test at the time of preparing the living will. The result of this can be recorded on the document. (See Appendix 7 for how to conduct the test.) If the patient's score is <22 this is evidence of mental impairment, and in these circumstances it might be unwise to co-operate with drafting any living will. Another way to augment the judgement that the patient is of sound mind, is to have a contemporaneous video recording of the elderly patient making his living will—ideally showing him to be in full executive control.

- Could the relatives bring unfair pressure to bear on the old person to sign a living will with which he does not fully agree? This is one of the chief advantages of having the patient's own doctor as an essential ingredient of a living will. He is the person most likely to be the trusted advocate of the patient, and is likely to know of sources of unwanted pressure. However, it is recognized that this is not a foolproof system. If there is any suspicion of unwanted pressure being brought to bear, the general practitioner is advised not to be a party to the will.

- Could the general practitioner himself bring unfair pressure to bear in the drawing up of a living will? It would be wrong to rely entirely on the honesty of all members of the profession. One way to avoid this problem would be to have a third party involved in the drawing up of the living will. This might be another doctor, or, better still, a vicar or lawyer. However, one does not want the process of making a living will to become too complicated—otherwise people will think that the reassurance of having a living will is beyond their reach and budget (particuarly if lawyers become involved).

- How is a living will revoked? The details of revocation will depend on the local circumstances prevailing when the will is drawn up. It is probably wise to designate one copy of the will the master copy, which can be revoked or added to, so that the possibility of having conflicting wills of apparently equal authority is avoided.

- What happens if the will directs the doctor to do something of question-able legality? Clearly a will cannot have force to compel a doctor to perform an illegal act. But if the act is of uncertain legal status, it is desir-able that legislation be drawn up to protect the doctor from legal proceedings in unclear areas in which he is acting according to the instruc-tions of a living will. In some states in America such legislation already exists (see Age Concern 1988).

The attention paid here to living wills may seem to be over-emphasized, and because their legal status is uncertain in the UK, all discussion might appear rather academic. In some communities the issue does not arise, but our own experience is that an increasing number of our patients are spontaneously raising these matters in consultations, or sending us such living wills through the post, to be kept in their medical records. Now that these have started to arrive, we need to know about them, how to help patients to draft them effectively, what their problems are, and how to protect ourselves and our patients from possible litigation.

In our own practice we do not think it is wise to disseminate information about living wills very widely. This is because the idea may be picked up by hearsay and distorted so that it looks as though the doctor were advocating euthanasia. If, however, as the result of publicity elsewhere a patient approaches us then we are happy to discuss the matter.

How valuable are old people?

Another area of ethical interest in geriatric aspects of general practice is encapsulated in the two questions: *'Are old people worth less than young people?'*—and: *'Who has more right to the limited resources of modern health care: the old person who has paid most towards them (via taxes) or the young adult who has paid nothing but stands to lose more?'* These questions are raised when there is pressure on resources, for example in coronary care, renal dialysis, intensive care heart transplants, and most other expensive high-technology medicine. (Note: this discussion concerns biological rather than chronological age.)

Let us take these questions in order. Let us not look at what people say in the comfort of an armchair (e.g. 'All lives have the same value, which is invariable, and remains constant'). Let us study how society answers these questions in its actions. We do not admit very old patients to that apotheosis and paragon of late twentieth-century medicine: the Coronary Care Unit. Why not? We used to offer ourselves platitudes such as 'Old people would not respond to the treatment: there is no evidence of real benefit to these patients'. This line of argument is becoming increasingly untenable. For example it is probable that the elderly are those who are most likely to benefit from thrombolytic therapy after acute myocardial infarction (as shown in the ISIS-2 trial, 1988). The older you are, the more certain the benefit (and the greater the risks, too, of course). Perhaps the reason is that we want to see our ideal world populated by ideal patients: young, attractive, verbal, intelligent, and sexually competent. If we fill up these lovely clean beds with incontinent old people, what will happen to our self-image? If we allow our all-pervading geriatric patients to penetrate even our central citadel of Coronary Care— then surely modern medicine will have started strangling itself with its own catheters? We do not generally articulate these conscious or unconscious thoughts because our self-image is not so simple. Our ideal patient may be young and successful, but our ideal doctor is all-loving, and unbiased by trivialities of age, sex, colour, or type of illness in those who are his patients. (Significantly, this ideal doctor is probably old and wise, not young and intelligent.) Once we become used to airing our attitudes about our elderly patients, we may come closer to shrugging off the malign influence of these forbidden thoughts, perhaps enabling us to accept our elderly patients more as they are. If we do so, we still have to say why we do not admit them to Coronary Care. If we abandon our malign attitudes, the only reason left is that we cannot afford to admit everyone to Coronary Care. Old people cost too much. Are we happy with this conclusion? Even if we had infinite resources and we turned the whole world into one glorious Coronary Care Unit we would still question the position of an elderly patient in such a Unit. Is it not rather tasteless or even morally destructive to try and prevent death at all costs and in all patients? Should not our old patients learn when to die? Coronary Care for everyone might have the effect of inducing death phobia in us all. We might spend all our energies trying to avoid the only certain thing in our world: a tragic (but predictable) position for modern man to find himself in. If we adopt our earlier principle ('If the patient's views are known, comply with them'), we should ask the patient what he or she wants. We should then telephone the hospital and ask if there is a bed on the Coronary Care Unit (if this is what the patient wants). If there is only one bed left, we might find ourself telling the patient that we think it should be kept for a younger patient. This may be a positive influence by encouraging altruism and a denial of death phobia—but it is not known if these sort of thoughts are helpful to the patient in acute illness. If the patient says: 'I am not going to be altruistic: I've paid for all this modern medicine through a lifetime of paying taxes. I deserve this scarce resource more than anyone else'—what should we say? In the acute stage there is no way for a patient to enforce his perceived rights. It is instructive to speculate that if he survives, his energies may, for example, be usefully directed towards influencing politicians to provide more health care.

Another argument to consider here is that society might decide, in the presence of limited resources, that if a patient has had a 'good innings' he or she should not expect expensive, life-saving medical interventions. We believe that this is a dangerous argument, and we note with satisfaction that the phrase 'He has had a good innings' is usually only used by doctors *after* the death of one of their patients, in order to comfort the family. If the expression is used before death, it would become very difficult to know what to say to patients who said that they were only just beginning to enjoy life at eighty. Other patients might be tempted to maximize their symptoms in their middle years, so that they could claim that they had *not* had a good innings when they reached some specified age. (What age? Who should specify it?) Also, where private medicine co-exists alongside state-run medicine it would seem unbearably unjust to deny one patient life-saving treatment, while his rich brother pays for far less medically valuable treatment in the private sector. One would have great difficulty with the doctor–patient relationship in these circumstances, and for this reason alone it is probably wise for decisions about making treatment unavailable to those who have had a good innings to be left to politicians who are safely out of the clinical arena.

5 Entering the minds of elderly people by the back door

We are all used to entering other people's minds by their front door—through their eyes and ears—and we are all too aware of the inadequacy of this route to knowledge. What is it like to grow old, and how do old people adapt to their changing capacities and cope with life? These are the central questions of gerontology: and only gerontologists know how to enter the mind by its back door—i.e. through the psychobiology of its concepts. We need to know about what gerontologists are up to, not because such knowledge will tell us what to prescribe in difficult cases, but because to understand is to forgive, and if we are not forgiving of the failures and foibles of the old we will hardly ever be able to help them (although this will not stop them being generous with their help and understanding of *us youngsters*).

Let us start with some uncharitable and by no means universally true observations about elderly people—and let us try to explain them:

1 Old people seem to be slow-witted.
2 Old people do not seem to know what is going on around them.
3 The conversation of old people often appears dead or wooden—with long monologues which are impossible to interrupt.
4 Old people seem very fond of digressing (?or regressing) to the very distant past and seem unable to take account of recent developments.
5 Old people's stories and anecdotes all too often turn out to be unamusing.

How can we ascribe meaning to phrases such as the psychobiology of the mind's concepts? Here is an example, starting with the observation that old people tend to forget the names of things, and can spend a lot of time with a word on the tip of their tongues. To account for this we suppose that the mind is like a dictionary in which the old person is trying to look something up, and in which some of the entries are written in faded ink, and some have been deleted. At first this sort of speculation and analogizing about the mind seems rather vacuous or self-obviously true. The point about gerontology is that it formally tests this sort of model—like this. If the mind is a dictionary in which you look things up, then people with the biggest dictionaries (i.e. the widest vocabularies) should take the longest to find a little-used but well-known word like 'frog'. Just the opposite is found to be true: those with the largest vocabularies name objects fastest. Deletions slow you down. So processing is not a linear or *sequential* activity. The awesome speed of thought as it swoops simultaneously from many buttresses at once in the great cathedrals and temples of the mind is only achievable by *parallel* processing, and the agonizing slowness of the decaying mind is interpretable in terms of a shortage of functioning buttresses (or nodes), with, in consequence, ruined choirs and collapsing naves which block the passage of thought. A node is a decision point, and how to get from a picture of leaping amphibian to the word 'frog' depends on using well-worn tracks through nodal networks of some complexity. The question now is: Are your nodal networks intact and how well worn are the tracks between them? If one node gets damaged or becomes non-operational, what are the collaterals like?

How does their decaying mind affect the lives of elderly people? Unadjusted performance IQ test scores fall sharply with age (Salthouse 1985), and with this comes much slower processing of information. Because of inevitable (p. 83) hearing loss it is harder for older people to remember what has just been said. This is thought to be because all the mind's free time is taken up with processing rather than with rehearsal of information. Rehearsal works as follows: if you catch a glimpse of the telephone number you want in the directory, and it is rather a long one, you repeat it over and over to yourself consciously or unconsciously, silently, or, even more effectively, out loud. But if it takes you a long time to process the number in the first place, you may arrive at the telephone without rehearsal—and misdial the number. Young people remember associations between auditorily presented pairs better than when the pairs are presented visually: *but in the elderly, just the reverse is true*. (Rabbitt 1989). If you cannot unconsciously rehearse material, you cannot remember what has just been said—and this explains why some elderly people are such unrewarding conversation partners. As Virginia Woolf so acutely observed, it is very difficult to share a good joke with a deaf person: there can be no *sotto voce* asides; and repeated punch-lines have no punch.

A clever person may be able to compensate for the ravages which age brings—by processing information faster than average, and by attending to peripheral cues as to what is going on. A less clever person may simply choose not to follow a long, devious, but boring story, and so gain for himself a reputation of being aloof and unfriendly. This may lead others to shun him, and as his practice at conversation using a defective sensorium dwindles, what started out as an unjustified reputation may quickly become all too justified. As Professor Rabbitt has said (1988):

If you are slow to decode what has just been said, or cannot integrate contributions from several speakers, it becomes hard to be witty or apposite. Your best remarks will usually be formulated too late. Rapid interjections may reveal embarrassing lapses of comprehension. Silence may seem morose and unfriendly. Continuous smiling is unenjoyable, and has dubious effects. If you seem pleasant as well as bewildered, officious help may be thrust upon you. In this no-win situation conversational habits which are sometimes classified as symptoms of egotistical personality defects, to which the elderly are particularly prone, may actually be no more than sad strategies of desperation. Forcing frequent disjunctions of topic may disconcert your company, but at least saves you from being judged morose, from a boring struggle to respond to what has been said, or from appearing much more stupid than and disorientated than you are. Monologuing may be boring for your audience, but it is much less so for you, and has the great advantage that you neither have to hear, nor to remember, what others have said.

Just what does it mean to say that clever old people may be able to mitigate the effects of ageing by using peripheral cues effectively? Here is a description of an experiment by Jocelyn Bryan which directly addresses this point. He measured IQs in a group of people aged between 50 and 79 years old, and showed them a series of newspaper-style photographs for 15 seconds—chosen because each one held more information than was obviously the case from looking just at each picture's central protagonist. Extra cues to the picture's meaning were, for example, from clothing and vegetation. After inspecting the photographs the subjects were immediately asked two types of questions: one type required simple recall of concrete detail; the other required *inferences*. It was found that older people failed to use even the most obvious cues, which led to quite unexpected distortions of the pictures' meanings. What seems to be lost is not the knowledge of the external worlds which enables us to interpret pictures, but rather the ability to relate new information to pre-existing complex knowledge structures, and, crucially, to make non-obvious associations between disparate events which allow us to make sense of incomplete sequences.

This ability to form non-obvious associations has been looked at in the following experiment. Elderly people were stratified by IQ and age and were asked to generate as many single-word associations to descriptive titles such as 'a meal in a restaurant' or 'a wedding'. Not surprisingly, older, less clever people, thought of fewer associations—even though there was no time-limit set on the task. The next phase of the experiment consisted in showing these newly-generated associations to a second group of people—again stratified according to IQ and age. The task of this second group was to say if they thought that the pairs presented (e.g. 'wedding' and 'ring') were associated or not. They were told that there were no correct answers, and that the experimenters were simply interested in their subjective thoughts. They were also told that responses would be timed, and they were asked to give an opinion as quickly as possible. Older people were not nearly so agile as others in saying 'Yes' to 'rare' associations.

The above analysis seems to go some way to explaining our first three observations about elderly people: what about the fourth—that of regression to the very distant past? That this does indeed happen has been shown in recent experiments in which volunteers aged from 50 to 86 were asked to recall incidents of any type from the first, second, or most recent third of their lives (Rabbit 1988). In the healthy elderly, very few incidents were recalled from the earliest period—but in those who were institutionalized and showed some evidence of cognitive impairment those few events which could be recalled all came from the first period. Interestingly, that they were institutionalized may be as important as the cognitive deficit in this regard. In a third group of people, who were institutionalized because of chronic physical disease but whose minds were cognitively intact (they remembered almost as many events as the normal group), it was found that they remembered almost as many incidents from their early years as from the recent past. We are led to the conclusion that regression to the past is an active strategy of the mind to mitigate the terminal tedium of institutionalized life. So the alternative to regression to the past may be far worse: an empty, passive mind—which we call dementia.

How can we analyse our fifth observation—that old people's stories and anecdotes all too often turn out not to be particularly funny? It is a relief to know that gerontologists do not yet have a device for quantifying humour (what would their unit of measurement be?—the Laurelandhardy, perhaps). This is not the chief difficulty in analysing such an evanescent quality as humour. Let us start with the observation that the quality of humour (as of all social interaction) depends on shared assumptions. The richer the network of shared assumptions, the richer becomes the possibility of humour. It was touching that a Mozart symphony was incorporated into the latest spacecraft to leave our solar system. Very few people would have thought of sending a joke on this journey through the vacancy of interstellar space in the hope that someone, somewhere would appreciate it. Similarly, on the long-stay geriatric ward, where, no doubt, the vacancies in interpersonal space are just as great, there is a corresponding miniscule chance of a joke being apprehended. Winthorpe has thrown some light on why this might be so (Rabbitt 1988). She has studied the way in which old people describe events from their past in normal conversation. Those with normal or high IQ test scores were good at offering complex grammatical structures and showed excellent management of sub-plots and supplementary details. With advancing years and falling IQ test scores, grammar becomes simpler and simpler, and descriptions become more and more generic with no richness of detail. For example, the person says 'I used to go sailing often'—without being able to recall an actual example of this activity. Perhaps these people have lost the ability to give rich accounts of their past through lack of practice. To test this hypothesis, these patients were all invited back, and an exact transcript of the previous interview was used in an energetic way to see if richer revelations could be accessed—but there was very little improvement. So this loss seems to be a fundamental ageing process—and when coupled with the slowness of processing information described earlier, we may well appreciate that the interactions on which humour depends are beyond the reach of many elderly minds.

The archetypal consultation with an old person

It is traditional to analyse consultations in terms of tasks, aims, and objectives (i.e. tasks defined; causes defined; exploration of patient's ideas and expectations; consideration of, at-risk factors and continuing problems; achieving appropriate actions, shared understandings, and patient involvement—and so on). To get to the heart of a geriatric consultation something a bit more subtle is needed in addition to all this—as the following analysis aims to demonstrate. We have chosen to explore the simplest of interactions: a visit by a (genuine) patient to request a repeat prescription. In this case we can record the patient's thoughts almost *verbatim*, because, uniquely in our experience, the patient had lost the ability to internalize her thoughts—which came out as very quiet speech, which, luckily, she could not hear because she was partially deaf. (This phenomenon has its counterpart in childhood, where we know that some children, when learning to read, can only ever read aloud—and this process of internalization can be long delayed.)

Dialogue (P = patient; D = doctor)	Patient's more or less conscious thoughts	Doctor's more or less unconscious thoughts	Line No.
P 'Please may I have some more of my tablets?'		Thank goodness that's all she wants.	1
D 'Yes, of course. Which tablets are these?'	Silly man: he never knows. [*Grits teeth*]		
P 'The ones for my chest, I think.'		Does she mean her angina or LVF or her antibiotics: Why can't she remember their names?—It's not much to ask.	5
D 'Were those the antibiotics? If so, they were a one-off thing.'		That might get me off the hook of having to distinguish her LVF from her angina.	10
P 'One off what?'	Why doesn't he talk sense?		
D 'You just take a course, and then that's it.'			15
P 'I think you said I would probably need to take them for the rest of my life or something . . .'		That won't be for very long if she can't even remember what her tablets are for.	
D 'Those are probably the ones for your heart.'	Stupid man: there's nothing wrong with my heart! I've had 14 children: how can there be anything wrong with my heart?		20
D 'Which is worse: your angina or your LVF?—Heart failure, I mean. No, not failure: it isn't failing, it's just what we call it, you know . . . .'		Damn! Why did I say that? Now I'm really making a hash of things: blinding her with abbreviations, and then making her think that her heart has failed. [*Doctor drives biro into desk.*]	25 30

Luckily the receptionist knew what the patient wanted and this consultation was saved from being a complete disaster. Nowhere is the communication gap more apparent than in this sort of consultation—where we recognize the following phenomena:

- The patient and the doctor both think that each other should be able to tell intuitively what the other one is getting at, or wants (lines 4–5).
- When this state of affairs does not come about, the doctor is not prepared for this. He is made angry and sarcastic (lines 16–18), and although this does not manifest itself directly in his behaviour or words, it might be at the root of what was an uncharacteristic mistake (line 25).
- Regression by the patient to the past (line 21)—with no insight into what has happened to her during the last half-century.
- Concrete thinking: line 13. 'One-off' is meant figuratively, but the patient takes it literally.
- Denial: line 21.
- Low threshold for exasperation: lines 3–4.
- Doctor minimizing contact with his patient: line 1.
- Emotional incontinence: patient—line 4; doctor (= J. M. L.)—line 30.

The purpose of bringing these phenomena to the attention of practitioners is so that he or she can recognize what is happening in consultations that are going wrong. The problem is that the patient and the doctor are responding to each other to and fro, tit for tat, like ping-pong players with a ball that is not bouncing properly. The doctor should consider disengaging himself, a process known as 'going meta' where 'meta' means going beyond, as in metaphysics (speculation going beyond the physical world) or meta-ethics (the art of choosing between competing theories of ethics—i.e. what lies beyond ethics) or meta-analysis (the science of finding universal but hidden truths by combining trials or analyses none of which individually reveals the truth in question). 'Going meta' means picking up the ball to see if it is cracked, rather than being trapped into hitting it harder and harder. It means operating in a third dimension to make sense of a muddled series of two-dimensional shadows. In the case above, it would mean saying something like 'We are not making much progress are we! Let me telephone your daughter.' Increasing frustration is the sign that you should 'go meta'—and a wry smile is the sign that you have accomplished this—as if you had said to yourself 'I know what's happening: it's all been described before, by that joke of a doctor on p. 41 of *Geriatric problems in general practice*—and now it is happening to me. What fun (!)—I'm in the real world: I'm doing geriatrics.' Of course, it is no coincidence that 'going meta' is associated with a smile. Humour is itself a process of finding a third dimension (hidden meaning) in something that seemed plain. It might be argued that a frustrating consultation is no laughing matter, and that when you have to get through a list of difficult patients as fast as possible because urgent visits are mounting up, the last thing you want to do is waste time laughing. The point of giving the above analysis in full is to show that humour is not a waste of time but a strategy for getting things done and keeping sane.

Part II Clinical geriatric medicine

6 Acute illness: repertoire of strategies

Many of the diseases and conditions which frequently affect the elderly are described in Chapter 7. The purpose of this chapter is to describe the aims and pitfalls in the management of acute problems: it is not intended as a catalogue of diseases and their management, but rather a programme of advice to maximize the repertoire of activities available to general practitioners when faced with an acutely ill elderly patient. Very often the leading symptom is simple enough, as would its management be—if the patient did not have other disabilities. The following example (based on a real case) illustrates this point.

Mrs RG is a widow living alone. Her main problem is immobility from chronic obstructive airways disease and arthritis. She usually manages with the help of her daughter who lives nearby. Today, however, she has called for a visit because of diarrhoea which has been worsening for the last four days. It turns out that her daughter has gone on holiday for a week, leaving some meals in her mother's fridge. As the days have been going by, the diarrhoea has begun spreading round the house. Mrs RG is frequently caught short on her way to her upstairs toilet. She has stopped eating, and is now drinking only small quantities of tea. The doctor calls and makes an assessment that things cannot go on for much longer like this. Apart from the insanitary conditions, the patient is starting to get dehydrated. The patient herself is also keen to be released from her misery, and would accept any reasonable proposal. What options are available to the general practitioner?

Admission to hospital

The first telephone call was to the nearby geriatric hospital. The house physician said that there were no female beds, but there might be one tomorrow. If it was urgent for today ... 'Please could you try the main hospital for acute admissions?' The second telephone call found a reluctant senior house officer who declined to accept the patient because of the diarrhoea 'I cannot admit a case of possibly infectious diarrhoea to the open ward ... We have got some very sick patients here, you know. Would you like to try the infectious diseases hospital?' The third telephone call is to the infectious diseases hospital. The admitting officer there rightly surmises that the patient's diarrhoea and its possibly infectious nature are only part of the problem. Understandably he does not want ... 'to get landed with a long-term geriatric problem, who probably has not got infectious diarrhoea anyway. If the patient has had diarrhoea for 4 days, why have you not done a stool sample? If the stool sample shows that the diarrhoea is infectious, we will admit her then.' In order to show his willingness, the general practitioner now arranges for a stool sample to be sent to the hospital. Unfortunately it just misses today's delivery so its analysis will be delayed—and, worse, prone to error because of the time delay. Then, in some desperation he rings up the consultant of the local chest unit under whose care the patient was last winter. He agrees to take the patient, provided there is a bed. He promises to ring back the beleaguered general practitioner. There is no speedy response, so the general practitioner starts afternoon surgery with the problem still quite unsolved. What other options does he have?

Admission to a local authority home for the elderly

A well-run home will occasionally have a bed available for emergency use. But such a home will be most unlikely to want to take an immobile, incontinent patient with diarrhoea. So it is probably not even worth ringing up to find out what the bed state is.

Admission to a private nursing home

Costs would be in the order of £250 a week. Mrs RG would also have to pay the cost of the ambulance journey (the ambulance service charges for journeys from one private address to another). Mrs RG owns her own house and has savings but only of a few thousand pounds. An admission to a nursing home would make a serious and unplanned dent in these savings. This is one reason for her reluctance to agree at once to admission to a nursing home. She is also of the opinion that in a nursing home one can be somewhat neglected, with not much more offered than three meals a day—which may not be suitable for one's condition. A third reason why she is reluctant to go to a nursing home is that '. . . once I'm in, will I ever come out again?' She knows that in hospital she will not be kept in a moment longer than is necessary. But in a nursing home she surmises that there is no real impetus towards discharge—and that there is a financial incentive *against* discharge. She would rather go to a small rest home where she would feel more in control of her future, and possibly be less institutionalized.

Admission to a rest home

The critical difference between a rest home and a nursing home is that there is no qualified nursing help available (so, for example, no possibility of injections or of prescribing anything but the simplest regimes) and the patient has to be mobile and continent and be able to look after herself. If Mrs RG was this good, she would not need admission at all. Are rest homes ever any help in the acute phase of a problem? The ideal acute problem where a rest home can be invaluable is depression. An old person living alone who gets a depression can become very isolated. If depression is severe drugs will usually be prescribed—but often not taken. The rest home can help ensure compliance. But, equally important, the best homes can provide a social ambiance which is as powerfully restorative as any antidepressant. They are often cheaper than nursing homes. Their main use is for convalesence, or simply as places to live.

Admission to an Abbeyfield Extra Care establishment

Abbeyfield is a charity set up to provide cheap accommodation for lonely elderly people. Their establishments are in receipt of grants from local authorities, private individuals, and other sources. Most function as simple rest homes, but a recent development is their 'extra care' activity. This usually takes place in a separate building, with rooms specially designed for immobile elderly patients. Quite a high level of care is available in theory, and they should certainly be able to manage a case of diarrhoea and incontinence, particularly if it is likely to be transitory. In practice, what an extra care establishment can cope with depends very much on the staff available—and in our own area this is a real problem. Mrs RG's doctor decides to try the local extra care Abbeyfield. He is told that it is too late to arrange anything today, but one of the patients currently being looked after is about to be 'discharged' back to an ordinary Abbeyfield establishment tomorrow afternoon. 'Would this be all right?' As it is the first offer of help Mrs RG's doctor has had after a large number of abortive telephone conversations he at once accepts, knowing he and Mrs RG still have 24 hours to get through. What options are available to help here?

Looking after Mrs RG at home

The first need is for a commode, which may be collected from the local hospital's porters if the home loans department is closed. The next need is for help in the house. A number of possibilities are available depending on local circumstances.

Relatives and neighbours   The whole crisis in the life of Mrs RG has arisen because her daughter has gone off on holiday—and her neighbours are unwilling or unable to help. Luckily the daughter has left a telephone number where she can be contacted. Surely the simplest thing is to telephone her, explain the situation, and encourage her to return to look after her now ill and dehydrated mother. Mrs RG's doctor decides that this is unfair. Mrs RG's daughter has spent months planning this holiday, and it will be the only time she can get away for the rest of the year, because the school holidays are ending. It may be necessary to inform the daughter if the clinical condition deteriorates—but only when a firm plan has been made, so that the daughter does not feel a moral pressure to curtail her holiday.

Volunteer sitters   These volunteers are sometimes able to come and be with an elderly person during times of difficulties—but often the agency needs a day's warning. It is certainly worth asking.

Twilight and night district nurses   Some health authorities have these available, along with a message desk which is manned 24 hours a day. The nurses ring in at specified times and pick up messages. In the case of Mrs RG their chief use would be to go along at bedtime and to make sure that the help you have arranged is actually working. They are *not* able to spend a prolonged time in the patient's home—because they will have other patients to attend to during the night. The great advantage of this service is its easy accessibility, and its suitability for use in emergencies. These nurses are also in communication with the regular district/community nurses, so messages can be passed on, and continuity of care is good.

Private domiciliary nursing agencies   These are also suitable for use in emergencies. For a fee of, say, £6 an hour a nurse can come in for any specified period—continuously (in shifts) or just at pre-arranged times. This gives a great feeling of security for relatives and the patient. It will be much cheaper for Mrs RG than a nursing home, because she will only be paying for what she gets. At nursing homes it is usually the practice for the patient to have to pay for *any* part of a working week during which he or she is a resident. So if Mrs RG was to go to a nursing home for a day before the Abbeyfield extra care bed becomes available, it would cost her some hundreds of pounds.

As Mrs RG has some savings, this is what her doctor deems to be the best interim solution. He rings the domiciliary nursing agency and gives clear instructions about the priorities of caring for Mrs RG. He concentrates on getting regular clear fluids drunk during the night, and arranges for the nurse to pick up a prescription for some codeine phosphate from surgery before she visits the patient. He ensures that the nurse knows how to contact him (or his partner on call) should the need arise.

Next day, Mrs RG telephones the surgery to say that she is feeling somewhat better, and is now no longer incontinent, as she can use the commode comfortably. The agency nurse has cleared up the mess at home, and she now feels that she can cope at home (without the agency nurse), if the district nurse could look in. Her doctor arranges this, and also undertakes to have a visit from the twilight nurse, to ensure that the arrangements are working, and that dehydration continues to be reversed. After discussion with the patient, the general practitioner decides not to tell the daughter of her mother's illness, until she returns. Mrs RG is keen that her daughter should not be put to unnecessary worry, and the general practitioner is now fairly confident that he does not have a mortal illness on his hands.

The above example serves to illustrate the importance of the general practitioner's local knowledge in optimizing the care of his elderly patients. In this case the normal channels of referral within the NHS proved fruitless. This may occasion much debate as to the origin of this perceived failure. But this will not be uppermost in the mind of the general practitioner as he is trying to arrange the care that his patient desperately needs. Privately, he may disagree with using the patient's own resources to provide the health care she needs, but if she is willing and there appears to be no alternative our hands are tied. In our own area, vast sections of the care of the elderly have already been privatized out of the NHS. The long-stay geriatric beds in our hospital have mostly been converted into acute beds, with their throughput depending crucially on the presence of privately run nursing homes and rest homes, so that the frail elderly can be discharged at the earliest safe opportunity, without having to wait for improvement to allow independent existence. The great advantage of this system is that admission to the geriatric hospital is now very much easier than before this system came into operation—so stories of refused hospital admission are much rarer now. The disadvantages of such reliance on the private sector is that what goes on inside nursing homes and rest homes is uncontrolled, unmonitored, and subject to much more variation than what goes on in hospital.

The financial aspects of relying on the private sector are not so bad for the patient as might first be thought. If the patient has little in the way of savings, local authority payments and an attendance allowance can go a long way to meeting the cost of care.

Other methods of optimizing acute care

The sphere of management has dominated our thinking on geriatric care. How do you manage depression, loneliness, dementia, hypothyroidism, or pneumonia?—to name five of the giants that stalk the corridors of our old people's homes. We take it for granted that diagnosis is not the chief problem: the problem lies in what to do once the diagnosis has been made. Let us test this assumption. Here is a list of examples from our own practice where we freely admit we are open to diagnostic error—and where diagnosis is the chief problem and management is enormously simplified once the diagnosis has been made.

Pulmonary embolism versus *myocardial infarction*

As a general rule of thumb whenever you diagnose myocardial infarction, ask yourself the question: *Could this be a pulmonary embolism?* This diagnosis is hard to make unless it occurs in the classical post-operative setting. Both myocardial infarction and pulmonary embolism cause chest pain, dyspnoea, cyanosis, and shock. The more specific features of a pulmonary embolism are hard to elicit: a loud pulmonary component to the second heart sound ($P_2\uparrow$) and a pleural rub. The ECG rarely contributes to the diagnosis, although it is worth looking for the classical (though rare) signs: Lead I, prominent S wave; Lead III, large Q wave and inverted T wave; V1–V4, T wave inversion. Similarly the chest X-ray will often look normal. There may be decreased vascular markings—but this may well be hard to diagnose on a domiciliary film (which, in any case, is a practical possibility for only a minority of general practitioners). Perhaps the best pointer to the diagnosis is evidence of a DVT. Failing this, consider the diagnosis of pulmonary embolism whenever it is clear that the patient has sustained *some* cardiorespiratory insult—but cardiac enzymes and ECGs are non-specific.

Stroke versus *subdural haemorrhage*

This differential diagnosis is particularly difficult in the elderly because trauma only needs to be very mild to produce a subdural haemorrhage, as the bridging veins between cortex and venous sinuses are particularly vulnerable because of brain shrinkage. Furthermore, even significant trauma—which would have provided a vital clue in the history—is all too often forgotten (brain shrinkage, again). The key to the diagnosis is to have a high level of suspicion, and to refer promptly anyone with a fluctuating level of consciousness *before* waiting for focal signs such as unequal pupils.

Fits versus *faints*

The key point here is to ask exactly how the episode started—and then to spare no effort in getting an accurate story from a witness. Nevertheless, witnesses are notoriously unreliable, being quite capable of subconsciously confabulating such vital features as clonic spasms if this is what they expect to see. Find out what position the patient was in when he or she began to feel bad. How much warning was there. A vertical posture (especially when stressed by hunger or heat) with a gradually blanking out of the field of view strongly suggests a faint. Whereas if there is an aura followed by focal features at the start of the attack, epilepsy is a much more likely diagnosis. Also pay attention to what happens after the attack. If there is a period of unilateral weakness (Todd's paresis), or a period of confusion or sleepiness, the diagnosis of epilepsy is supported. In the elderly tongue-biting is still a useful sign of epilepsy—but incontinence less so.

Acute asthma versus *acute pulmonary oedema*

If you are faced by a collapsed patient who is centrally cyanosed and wheezing with bilateral crepitations, it may take a considerable time to amass enough evidence to say whether the cause is acute asthma or acute pulmonary oedema, and the patient may well die before you can reach a definitive diagnosis. In these circumstances, have no hesitation in treating both at once with oxygen, and parenteral diamorphine, frusemide, terbutaline, and steroids (± a vasodilator). If the clinical state is not too desperate you may have time to approach a diagnosis. If the cause is pulmonary oedema there may be signs of pre-existing or current heart disease (pulsus alternans, large heart, gallop rhythm, JVP↑, hepatomegaly—and diuretic tablets found by the bedside). In acute bronchial asthma, look for pulsus paradoxus—and bronchodilators by the bedside.

Cardiogenic shock versus *hypovolaemic shock*

This distinction is hard enough in younger, fitter patients—but in the elderly it is doubly difficult because the history may be quite misleading, and the physical signs conflicting. For example, the patient may have had a large myocardial infarction, but have felt no pain. Or he may be bleeding fast enough to make his angina worse—but without a tell-tale tachycardia because he is taking a beta-blocker. It is important to try and make the correct diagnosis—and often it will be appropriate to refer those with hypovolaemic shock, while those with cardiogenic shock may be assumed to have had a myocardial infarction (if there are no unusual features), and are managed according to different priorities. Dissection of the ascending aorta (e.g. with retrograde spread causing cardiac tamponade) may be a possible diagnosis to make if arm pulses and blood pressure are unequal. Tamponade is suggested by Beck's triad: a rising pulse, a falling blood pressure, and a small, quiet heart. A rectal examination can be very helpful in determining the cause of shock. Once melaena is found, the course of action is usually clear.

Acute back pain versus *acute loin pain*

Patients often find it difficult to point accurately to the site of either lumbar or loin pain—particularly if they are old and arthritic—and hence are likely to attribute all pain in that area to the lumbar spine. When in doubt, examine the urine. We use a portable microscope for this purpose—which, on occasion, gives very valuable information. The techniques are described elsewhere (Longmore 1986). Red cells can also be detected using foil-wrapped (hence long shelf-life) *N-Labstix®*.

Organizational aspects

The diagnosis and management of acute medical problems in the elderly is frequently a time-consuming task. If we can engage in forward planning, it is possible to look after a surprising number of very difficult illnesses in the home. In our practice we have, on any given day, an emergency doctor for acute visits, who alternates with the clinic/surgery doctor. This arrangement means that difficult visits do not have to be squeezed in between surgeries, but can be given the time they deserve. This enables households to be transformed into high-dependency units, with oxygen, intravenous fluids (drips), and injections, and regular monitoring of vital signs can be accomplished (e.g. through regular visits by the district nurse). In the surgery we have the ability to carry out all the commonly required laboratory tests (such as haemoglobin, total white cell count, differential white cell count (and film), plasma potassium, cardiac enzymes, and other biochemical parameters such as drug therapeutic monitoring (using test reagent strips and solid state assays from Ames laboratories and their remarkable but somewhat temperamental *Seralyser-III*®. These organizational aspects have enabled us to look after patients who have decided to remain in their own homes—with diagnosis such as pulmonary embolism, myocardial infarction, unstable angina, pneumonia, status epilepticus, respiratory failure, malignant hypertension, and septicaemia.

7 Common diseases and conditions of the elderly*

Abuse of the elderly

The Eastman definition (Harris 1988): Misuse of power resulting in a reduction of the quality of an elderly person's life. Eight types have been identified:

- Nutritional deprivation
- Maladministration of drugs
- Verbal abuse
- Financial abuse
- Sexual abuse
- Failure to attend to health needs
- Isolation, confinement, or restraint (e.g. in Buxton chairs)
- Assault

Unrelenting stress is the chief association: not social class. People with dementia and Parkinsonism are most vulnerable, as the fluctuating nature of their disabilities can make it seem that the elderly person is being wilfully difficult. Most carers are relieved to be asked about their feelings of aggression—but only about 20 per cent wish that the elderly person in their care could be looked after full-time in a residential home. Two-thirds of carers admit to losing their tempers, and 20 per cent admit to having hit the person in their care—the same proportion who report having been hit themselves by the elderly person.

Isolation and ignorance of financial support and carers associations might be important causes of aggression.

Some institutions inevitably abuse the elderly because of the way they work—e.g. no privacy; no flexibility in arrangements (e.g. evening meal never later than 5 p.m.).

No equivalent of the 'Place of Safety Order' so useful in paediatric practice exists: indeed, the hospital (the usual 'Place of Safety') may simply perpetuate or augment the abuse. Other countries (e.g. Germany) have systems of written contractual obligations (rights and duties of *both* parties).

If abuse is suspected, the only system of redress in the UK is section 47 of the National Assistance Act.

* The problems are listed in alphabetical order.

Anaemia

Although most doctors will accept as normal a lower haemoglobin in older people than they would in younger patients, there is no logical reason for this to be the case. For practical purposes, however, it is often necessary to adopt a cut-off point below which further investigation is necessary, and a level less than 12 g/dl of blood should raise thought about further investigation, as also should any consistent downward trend, even if the level is above this. It is all too easy to dismiss a low haemoglobin as being an expected finding in an old person and deny them the opportunity of appropriate treatment for an underlying condition which might well improve the quality of their life. As is usually the case, the assessment of an anaemia is facilitated by subdividing the anaemias on the basis of the mean corpuscular volume into microcytic, macrocytic, and normocytic types.

Microcytic anaemia   This is the commonest anaemia of old age and is nearly always due to iron deficiency. It is best confirmed by checking the serum iron and total iron-binding capacity or ferritin levels, but if these are found to be normal it is necessary to consider other possibilities, in particular a sideroblastic anaemia, or more rarely a thalassaemia, and in these circumstances hospital referral is necessary. When detecting an iron-deficiency anaemia the first step in an older person is to exclude dietary inadequacy. This may be indicated in the history, or there may be other biochemical evidence of malnutrition. Gastric irritation and consequent blood loss is another frequent finding, especially when a patient is taking certain drugs, such as aspirin and the non-steroidal anti-inflammatory analgesics. Gastro-intestinal neoplasms and peptic ulcers also frequently turn out to be the cause of this type of anaemia. GI tract blood loss may be confirmed by finding positive faecal occult blood, but this test can be misleading, and if a gastro-intestinal cause for the anaemia is suspected, barium studies and possibly endoscopy are indicated—after a careful abdominal and rectal examination. Although a gastric neoplasm is unlikely to be surgically treated, other conditions such as peptic ulceration respond well to treatment. If it is not possible or appropriate to arrange these tests, then it is reasonable to prescribe a course of iron and observe the results. In the case of a suspected peptic ulcer a trial of appropriate therapy may well prove beneficial. Other causes of iron deficiency include blood loss from other sites, malabsorption, and haemolysis.

Macrocytic anaemia   Vitamin B_{12} and folate deficiency are the commonest cause of a macrocytic anaemia in elderly people. Folic acid deficiency may be associated with some drugs, e.g. phenytoin and co-trimoxazole. In theory, before attributing a macrocytic anaemia to a deficiency of one of these, it is necessary to confirm the presence of megaloblastic change in the bone marrow. This is so because there are other causes of macrocytosis, including alcohol ingestion, liver disease, thyroid disease, vitamin C deficiency, and even a high reticulocyte level, since immature red blood cells are larger than the normal corpuscle. If, however, an estimation of the serum B_{12} or folate reveals one of these to be low, it is often reasonable to prescribe the appropriate replacement therapy and monitor the result (ask specifically for reticulocyte enumeration: a brisk reticulocyte response—e.g. 10 per cent—indicates a satisfactory response). If it is decided that both B_{12} and folate should be given, the B_{12} should be started first and a loading dose given as well. The folic acid can be prescribed subsequently. The reason for this ordering is that if folic acid is given alone, subacute combined degeneration of the cord may be precipitated.

If there is B_{12} or folate deficiency it is necessary to consider the possibility of malnutrition due to an inadequate diet or malabsorption, and if appropriate, investigate accordingly. Barium studies and endoscopy are occasionally necessary, especially if there is a history of gastrointestinal symptoms—since carcinoma of the stomach occurs more frequently in people with a history of pernicious anaemia. Also, Crohn's disease of the terminal ileum or another lesion here may well be interfering with the absorption of B_{12}. Less commonly, a barium meal and follow-through will reveal small bowel diverticula, which may also be responsible for B_{12} deficiency. It is, however, not appropriate to subject an older person to a barium meal simply because they have B_{12} deficiency, unless there is an additional indication to do so.

When following up a patient in whom pernicious anaemia has been confirmed, it is important to remember that there is an increased incidence of other autoimmune diseases, especially thyroid disorders, Addison's disease due to adrenal atrophy, rheumatoid arthritis, and diabetes mellitus.

Normochromic/normocytic anaemia   A normochromic/normocytic anaemia is usually a concomitant of chronic disease, the aetiology of which is often very difficult to elucidate. The most important to be alert to are: chronic renal failure, chronic infection, especially subacute bacterial endocarditis and tuberculosis, collagenoses, and malignancy. Occasionally, a normochromic normocytic picture is the result of a haemolytic process, in which case there will usually be other confirmatory evidence, such as an elevation of the urinary urobilinogen level and a film suggestive of haemolysis. There may also be signs of a reticulocyte response and an elevated serum bilirubin. Haemolysis is discussed further in the section on jaundice.

Arthritic complaints

The commonest causes of arthritis in the elderly are osteoarthrosis and rheumatoid arthritis, and in the case of the latter there is often a superimposed element of osteoarthrosis. Although touched on briefly elsewhere, each merits consideration in its own right.

Osteoarthrosis   The classical presentation of osteoarthrosis involves the complaints of pain, stiffness, and in some joints deformity. Inflammation in the usual sense is absent, but there may be an effusion and occasionally the joint may feel warm. In the latter case this is probably more frequently associated with local trauma than with the arthritis itself. Osteoarthrosis may also present in other ways, for instance the rupture of a Baker's cyst in the popliteal fossa, producing a clinical picture simulating a DVT, or in the more general sense of impaired ability to perform the activities of daily life. It is unrealistic to expect to confirm the diagnosis radiologically in every diseased joint. However, an X-ray should be considered necessary whenever the symptoms are atypical or the possibility of pyogenic arthritis is considered, or where the expected response to therapy is not forthcoming.

Treatment

In the initial stages many geriatricians prescribe simple analgesics, such as paracetamol, although this is considered inappropriate by some. Despite this many elderly patients appear to benefit from the pain-relief that is gained, and are not exposed to the more hazardous side-effects of the non-steroidal anti-inflammatory drugs. If a trial of simple analgesics is unsatisfactory, non-steroidal anti-inflammatory preparations should be prescribed, but the side-effects, especially dyspepsia, gastrointestinal-tract bleeding, and fluid and salt retention must not be forgotten.

Physiotherapy is the other mainstay of treatment. This can be carried out in the patient's home in those areas where there is a domiciliary physiotherapy service, or otherwise in a physiotherapy department or a day hospital. This should not be considered just remedial, but also of preventive value. Physiotherapy can play a major contribution in preventing muscle weakness and wasting associated with arthritis. The authors recognize that in some areas GPs only have access to physiotherapists for patients less than 65 years old. If this is the case, one possibility is to teach the patient to be his or her own physiotherapist.

More specific measures are sometimes necessary, depending upon the joints involved. In the case of the lower limb, dietary restriction in an obese patient may lead to significant weight loss and help relieve the symptoms of arthritis in the hip and the knee. Dietary measures unfortunately are often unsuccessful in the elderly. In the case of degenerative disease of the cervical spine a cervical collar is often beneficial, and it is not always appreciated that in many instances it should be worn at night as well as during the day. It is also important to remember that degenerative diseases of the cervical spine may result in cord compression. A lumbar corset may be necessary for degenerative changes in the lumbar spine.

Sadly many elderly patients are denied consideration of surgical relief of their symptoms simply because they are regarded as too old by their medical attendants, or the orthopaedic surgeons involved. It is extremely important to remember that biological rather than chronological age is the relevant factor, and in any patient in whom medical treatment has failed to alleviate the symptoms surgical intervention should be considered. This is particularly important for arthritis of the lower limbs, as loss of mobility may herald the end of independence for the patient concerned.

Rheumatoid arthritis   Rheumatoid arthritis infrequently arises for the first time in elderly patients, but it can often continue to flare-up in the later years, pursuing a course that began sometime in middle or earlier life. Most frequently, however, rheumatoid arthritis in the elderly is of the 'burned-out' variety associated with superimposed osteoarthrosis. Should it start in old age the symptoms and joint disease can be quite severe, but in general there are fewer erosions and nodules than in younger patients. In addition the systemic manifestations are usually less predominant than in younger patients, although there will usually be a high ESR and a normochromic, normocytic anaemia.

Treatment

It is important to avoid prolonged bed-rest in older patients if this is at all possible, and especially necessary to remember the possibility of contracture development, which may require the use of a splint for an inflamed joint.

The non-steroidal anti-inflammatory preparations are usually the mainstay of treatment, but do not forget their side-effects mentioned earlier. Note: phenylbutazone is now obsolete because of the hazard of aplastic anaemia and bone-marrow depression. If steroids are used it is essential to reduce the dose as soon as possible to 7.5 mg of prednisolone daily or less, in order to minimize the risk of steroid-induced side-effects.

Intra-articular injections must be performed with scrupulous attention to sterility as many elderly patients have an increased susceptibility to infection. Although it may be necessary to prescribe disease-modifying drugs such as gold therapy or penicillamine for rheumatoid arthritis in the elderly, these treatments are probably best reserved for hospital supervision, as the side-effects can be extremely toxic.

As in the case of osteoarthrosis, the physiotherapist plays an important part in treating patients with rheumatoid arthritis, but the occupational therapist is especially important in his or her role of helping the patient to overcome or come to terms with the difficulties experienced in activities of daily living.

When medical treatment is unsuccessful or a patient presents with a severely disorganized joint, an elderly patient should not be barred from consideration of a surgical procedure such as synovectomy or joint replacement.

Crystal arthropathies   Gout and pseudogout are not infrequently en-countered in the elderly. Gout is commoner in women, contrary to popular opinion, and it must not be forgotten that there may be an underlying blood dyscrasia as its cause. An elevated uric acid level alone does not confirm the diagnosis of gout, since this occurs commonly as a manifestation of drug therapy, especially with thiazide diuretics. The diagnosis is confirmed by discovering the characteristic crystal deposits in an effusion from the joint.

As in younger patients, gout is treated by resting the joint and prescribing a non-steroidal anti-inflammatory agent initially, and occasionally colchicine. For longer-term maintenance treatment, allopurinol rather than uricosuric drugs is probably best, and in the first two or three months of prescription it is wise to give a prophylactic dose of a non-steroidal anti-inflammatory agent such as indomethacin to counteract the acute attacks that may be pre-cipitated. Avoid salicylates and uricosuric drugs until the acute attack is over. If allopurinol is prescribed, monitor plasma uric acid, so that the minimum of this quite expensive drug is used—and the risk of side-effects is least (hepatotoxicity, hypertension, headaches, and hair loss). Allopurinol has important interactions with some cytotoxic agents—increasing their toxicity.

The diagnosis of pseudogout is often made radiologically with the discovery of chondrocalcinosis on an X-ray of a joint, usually the knee. A definitive diagnosis, however, as in the case of gout, relies upon finding the appropriate crystals in an effusion from a joint. In this case calcium pyrophosphate crystals are found. Pseudogout in the elderly is usually unassociated with other conditions, although both hyperparathyroidism and haemochromatosis may occur in association with it. These therefore should be considered and it is traditional to exclude these in any patient in whom chondrocalcinosis has been found (but as management may not be changed this practice is very much open to question).

The treatment of acute attacks of discomfort in a patient with pseudogout is the same as in the case of a patient with gout. Often, however, aspiration of an effusion will abort the attack for reasons that are obscure.

Backache

Confusion often exists about the causes of backache in the elderly—since osteoporosis is a common finding and discomfort is commonly attributed to its presence. Osteoporosis on its own, however, probably rarely accounts for backache unless there is an accompanying crush fracture of one or more of the vertebrae. This cannot be satisfactorily diagnosed without an X-ray, even if there is typical girdle-like radiation of pain. It should be treated with analgesics, lumbar support, and physiotherapy. In the case of severe pain hospitalization or attendance at a day hospital may be necessary, but one should always remember that in the presence of a crush fracture other causes should be excluded, such as myeloma and secondary deposits. This is because the osteoporosis itself may not be responsible, since it is present in so many people without symptoms.

Other conditions which cause backache include osteoarthritis in the spine and the sacroiliac joints. Many people, however, have signs consistent with the diagnosis of early spinal osteoarthritis without experiencing any symptoms and so one has to think carefully before attributing a person's discomfort to this cause. When it is responsible for back pain, there is often a history of trauma and it may be the latter rather than the arthritis itself that is symptomatic. In the case of the sacroiliac joints the symptoms can often be relieved by local injection of local anaesthetic and/or hydrocortisone. Secondary deposits, especially from the lung, prostate, breast, and in myeloma, may cause back pain without vertebral collapse. It is important to look for the primary since in certain cases, e.g. breast and prostate, the patient may well be helped by hormone treatment. A useful pointer is that breast and prostatic deposits are often sclerotic, and in the case of prostatic carcinoma, a high alkaline and acid phosphatase indicates the probability of metastatic spread. Myeloma and occasionally a hypernephroma may be indicated by finding a very high ESR. Bone pain from metastatic deposits can often be relieved with prostaglandin inhibitors, e.g. indomethacin, but sometimes local radiotherapy is necessary.

Paget's disease may also cause backache, but will be apparent from an X-ray and can be further suspected in the presence of a very high alkaline phosphatase. Most commonly, however, backache is probably a result of soft-tissue disorders which are self-limiting and need treating only with analgesics and support. It must not be forgotten that pain may be referred to the back from an evolving abdominal aortic aneurysm or an intra-abdominal viscus, e.g. a peptic ulcer, gastric neoplasm, and pancreatitis; that infective conditions occasionally localize into and around the spine; and herpes zoster can present with pain before the rash occurs. Osteomalacia (see p. 116) can also be responsible for back pain, and is diagnosed with the usual radiological and biochemical investigations.

The management of back pain includes therefore a well-directed history, examination of the abdomen and breasts as well as the back—and an X-ray of the spine if symptoms persist or there are features suggesting a sinister cause. Laboratory investigation may then be organized on the basis of the radio-logical and other findings, if any. Should the discomfort persist, especially in the presence of weight loss or other evidence of systemic disease, referral for further investigation is necessary.

Cardiac failure

Mild heart failure is best treated with a small dose of a thiazide diuretic and potassium supplement or one of the combination preparations that includes a potassium-sparing component. In more moderately severe heart failure a loop diuretic such as frusemide and/or a vasodilator may be necessary. Loop diuretics require additional potassium supplementation or the concomitant use of a potassium-sparing agent. Loop diuretics are usually unnecessary in the longer term, however.

Severe heart failure is probably best treated in hospital, but where this is not practical the following approach will usually be helpful. Try to get a baseline weight recording. This can be a very useful marker of how therapy is going, and gives early warning of relapses. Bed rest is important and loop diuretics are often the mainstay. Venodilators such as isosorbide mono-nitrate may particularly relieve the symptoms of dyspnoea, whilst the arteriolar dilators such as hydralazine are more helpful in relieving fatigue, lethargy, etc. In the majority of cases venodilators are preferable. Sometimes it is necessary to use a combined arteriolar and venodilator approach, in which case the angiotensin converting enzyme inhibitors (ACE inhibitors) are probably now becoming the most widely used agent in older patients, particularly captopril and enalapril (see p. 150).

In the elderly, especially men, one has to remember that potent diuretics may precipitate urinary retention, and if this occurs temporary catheteriza-tion may be required. It is also important to remember that the successful resolution of severe heart failure should be followed by reducing and simplifying the therapeutic regime. It is rarely necessary to leave an old person on a maintenance dose of a loop diuretic.

Finally, the onset of heart failure, especially if it occurs acutely, should prompt a search for any underlying or exacerbating cause which is remediable (e.g. hyperthryoidism, anaemia).

Cerebrovascular accident

Having confirmed that a patient has suffered a stroke the next decision that must be made is whether or not they should be admitted to hospital. There are undoubtedly many people who have either a minor CVA or adequate home support who can be completely managed at home. Despite this it is the authors' opinion that the majority of people with a stroke should be admitted to hospital, at least initially. Domiciliary care can then be resorted to early on if this is appropriate. In a patient in whom domiciliary care is anticipated the following points should be assessed in every case.

1. Aetiology

It is essential to ensure that there is no treatable underlying cause which could lead to further episodes if not discovered and treated in time.

(a) Common cardiovascular conditions include:

Hypertension—but it must be remembered that a mild elevation of blood pressure may be the result and not the cause of the stroke.

Arrhythmias—which may lower cardiac output and also be responsible for systemic embolization.

Systemic embolization from valvular heart disease, a mural thrombus after a coronary, and large-vessel atheroma. Evidence for the latter may be found by listening for a bruit in the neck.

(b) Central nervous system—a tumour or space-occupying lesion will usually produce a gradual or slow onset. Other occasional catches in the elderly include Todd's paralysis after an epileptic attack, a subdural haematoma, and, less frequently, meningitis. The patient's history of epilepsy may not have been known, and the seizure may not have been witnessed. In theory a subdural haematoma should have fluctuating signs, but this is not always the case. The presence of meningism and a fever will usually indicate the possibility of meningitis, although blood in the cerebrovascular space produces a similar clinical picture.

(c) Giant cell arteritis—this occasionally presents with localizing neurological signs and should be suspected if the appropriate history can be elicited or the patient is known to have a high ESR.

(d) Diabetes mellitus—both hypo- and hyperglycaemia may be associated with localizing neurological signs and indicate the need for attention to the underlying problem.

(e) A high haemoglobin (polycythaemia)—e.g. associated with chronic hypoxaemia—may also cause strokes.

It can therefore be seen that there are a sufficient number of treatable underlying precipitating factors to warrant the admission of many patients with a stroke to hospital, even if the disability is in itself not an adequate reason for this. In any patient in whom domiciliary care was initially considered, the presence or suspicion of one of these conditions, or of any other condition that has not been mentioned but is in itself treatable, should lead to hospital referral unless it can be treated with the patient at home or it is considered that the time has come for the patient to be allowed to die gracefully and with dignity at home. Even this decision can be fraught with danger, however, since many patients recover when expected not to do so, and failure to direct prompt attention to the underlying illness, or later on to organize rehabilitation early enough in the recovery phase, may lead to a greater degree of eventual dependency. The key question (apart from the availability of hospital beds) is 'What does the patient want?'—and whether you have enough energy to exclude remedial causes by investigation at home. Often it is hard to decipher what the patient wants—but if his or her wishes are known, comply with them.

2. Determine the site of the lesion

Cerebrovascular damage in the elderly commonly occurs in the region of the internal capsule. Through this structure pass motor fibres, the majority to the other side of the body but in the case of those muscle groups with bilateral innervation, namely the trunk, limb girdles, and neck, to the ipsilateral side also. Sensory and autonomic fibres are also present in the internal capsule and lead to the sensory abnormalities and disturbance of autonomic function in the affected limbs. Fibres connecting with the extrapyramidal system are also present and it may be that damage to these is partly responsible for the alteration in tone and eventual onset of spasticity. Fibres from the optic radiation pass through the lateral wing producing a homonymous field defect, often a full hemianopia.

If the cerebral cortex is involved there will be flaccid weakness affecting flexor and extensor muscle groups equally, whereas in the internal capsule lesion there is usually hypertonicity of the flexors and abductors in the arms and of the extensors in the legs. Other indications of a cortical lesion are the typical picture of cortical sensory loss and speech problems, especially dysphasia.

A lesion of the brainstem will produce multiple signs because of the large number of vital structures crowded together in a small space. It is usually manifested by the involvement of cranial nerve nuclei affecting the ipsilateral side, since these fibres tend to cross high in the brainstem, and contralateral weakness in the limbs. Evidence of cerebellar involvement or vertigo also indicates a brainstem-territory lesion. Pontine haemorrhage should be suspected in a deeply unconscious patient with bilateral paralysis, small pupils, and a pyrexia. (Small pupils may also be caused by opiates and anticholinergic eye drops as used in glaucoma, and it is possible to be caught out by one of these if the possibility is not considered.)

It is necessary to identify the site of the lesion because of the relevance of this to the prognosis. Brainstem lesions in particular have a poor prognosis.

3. Consider the potential prognosis

In an individual patient it is often very difficult to know at the beginning what the outcome is going to be. In general, however, there are many points which may influence the outcome, and these include the site of the lesion as discussed above; the patient's conscious level—since the prognosis is worse in non-haemorrhagic lesions if the patient is unconscious; the functional level—since the outlook is better the greater the functional level initially; aphasia—since the absence of this indicates a favourable outlook; and parietal lobe damage—which is usually associated with poor functional recovery. In addition one needs to take into account the associated diseases, including those which might precipitate a further cerebrovascular event and those which may cause morbidity in their own right.

4. Further management

In the acute phase it is also necessary to assess carefully those factors which may prejudice the patient's survival, including the swallowing reflex and the state of hydration. Later, i.e. during the recovery period, it is important to check the following regularly: (i) urinary and faecal incontinence; (ii) pressure sores; (iii) deep venous thrombosis and pulmonary emboli; (iv) constipation; (v) hypostatic pneumonia, and (vi) contractures.

In theory these are all treatable or preventable sequelae and should be attended to as appropriate. It may well be necessary to supplement domiciliary rehabilitation by referring the patient to a geriatric clinic for consideration of additional rehabilitation, e.g. through the day hospital, after the acute phase is over and the patient has begun to return to normal life.

Finally, it is important to note that there is no objective evidence for any benefit in the long term following a completed stroke from the prescription of anticoagulants, aspirin, dipyridamole, dextran, or steroids. Each of these may be of prophylactic benefit in certain situations, e.g. anticoagulation in the presence of mitral stenosis and atrial fibrillation, but it is unlikely to affect a stroke which has already occurred. Antiplatelet measures, however, including low-dose aspirin, are now considered by many authorities to reduce the incidence of a CVA after TIA.

Useful advice for old people and their relatives

Coping with dysphasia

1 Talk a little more slowly than normal.
2 Use short sentences of simple construction but not childish language.
3 Avoid 'either . . . or' questions . . . try to ask questions which require yes or no.

4 Do not rush to finish sentences or supply words.
5 Supplement the spoken word with mime, for example, pointing to the object discussed or miming drinking a cup of tea. Try using drawings and pictures of everyday objects for the patient to point to.
6 Remember that the patient can often understand much more than he can say. Do not discuss sensitive matters in front of him.
7 Put important instructions in writing.
8 Ask the advice of speech therapists if the patient is in hospital or attends day hospital. While it is not clear what improvement speech therapists can bring about in this situation, there is no doubt that their role in improving morale and instilling the will to get better is one of their chief assets.

Confusion and dementia

It is often very difficult to be certain whether an elderly person is confused or demented. One has to differentiate the abnormal from normal mental ageing, and although this is often easier in the case of an acute confusional state, diagnosing early dementia is often far from easy. Dementia is a global impairment of intellectual ability, and it is important also to test for variables other than memory loss. Examples of these are temporal and parietal lobe function, including aphasia, e.g. pointing to a watch and asking what it is called, and then something a little more difficult like the watch strap and then the hand. This will indicate the presence of motor aphasia, whilst an indication of receptive problems can be gained from enquiring into the function of common domestic articles. Parietal lobe abnormalities can be elicited by asking the patient to raise their right or left hand, to touch their left knee with their right hand, or vice versa, to identify a coin or small object held in the hand, and to draw a square or a clock face. This is a much more sensitive way of ascertaining the presence of a dementing illness than merely relying upon a memory test.

It is also important to mention at this point that the pseudodementia of depression must always be considered if there are other signs indicating the possibility of a depressive illness.

Acute confusional states   The commonest cause is undoubtedly infection, especially of the respiratory or urinary tract. Endocrine and metabolic abnormalities are often responsible, including hyperglycaemia, drugs, (especially antiparkinsonian agents, hypnotics, sedatives, and antidepressants), nutritional deficiencies, especially B_{12} and possibly folate, and abnormalities of the urea and electrolytes. Two of these categories, namely myxoedema and nutritional deficiencies, tend to have a slower onset of action than is normally considered classical for an acute confusional state and are more likely to cause dementia, but on occasions have been noted to present with an apparently rapid onset. This may be because the patient has deteriorated without its being noted, until some event makes it more apparent.

Other causes include a cerebrovascular accident, a subdural haematoma, an intracerebral space-occupying lesion, a non-metastatic effect of neoplasm of the bronchus, and other physical problems, such as cardiac and respiratory failure.

It is important also to bear in mind the other causes of a more chronic dementing illness, since, as was mentioned earlier, these can apparently have an acute onset because of the way in which the problem presents.

Useful points for relatives

- Alzheimer's disease is a terminal illness. Nobody ever gets better from it. Most are dead within 7 years.
- It is good to start grieving for the loss of the demented person now. The person who you knew, for example as your parent or spouse, now no longer exists—but has been replaced by the person you now care for.
- Take every opportunity you can to talk about your predicament with other people in the same position. This is often just as useful as talking to professionals. The Alzheimer's Disease Society exists to put you in touch (UK phone number: 081 675 6557).
- Accept any offer of day-care for your relative. It will give you much-needed respite from the task of looking after your relative.
- Lock up any rooms in the house which you do not use. Your relative will not notice this restriction—and this may make your life much easier.
- Lock any drawers which contain important papers or easily-spoiled items. This will prevent the patient storing inappropriate things in them, such as compost from the garden, or worse.
- Remove locks from the lavatory—so he/she cannot get locked in.
- Normal sexual relationships will probably stop. Spouses should try not to fall into the trap of asking 'What's the matter with me?'
- Prepare yourself psychologically for the day when he/she no longer recognizes you. This can be a great blow, unless you prepare for it.
- Apply to Social Services for an Attendance Allowance, if appropriate.

Note: we do not envisage giving such stark advice to the carer the moment the diagnosis is made. Some groundwork needs to be done first. However, all the evidence (based on the wishes of the carers themselves) is that we tend to give this sort of advice far too late—if ever (Morgan 1989).

The initial step in diagnosis is to exclude infection, to check a patient's drugs and relate the onset of confusion to the duration of drug therapy, and then to screen for the other conditions, e.g. with the aid of a blood-sugar level, urea and electrolyte estimation, haemoglobin, white count and ESR, and any other investigation that seems appropriate as a result of the history and examination. If a cause is not found, or an illness is encountered which cannot be successfully treated at home, early referral to the geriatric service is necessary.

Chronic confusion/dementia   If this has been present for six months or so it is likely that the patient has an irreversible condition such as multiple infarct dementia or more commonly senile Alzheimer's disease. Despite this it is always necessary to exclude the treatable conditions (see below), rectification of which may lead to an improvement in the patient's mental abilities, although often the best that one can hope for is that the progress of the dementia will be arrested or retarded.

Senile Alzheimer's disease is the commonest cause of senile dementia. The other most commonly occurring condition is multi-infarct dementia, i.e. mental impairment resulting from a progression of small strokes. In theory, this condition is more likely if the deterioration has been step-wise rather than gradual, the patient has a history of hypertension, or there is evidence of vascular disease elsewhere. It is not always possible, however, to rely upon this evidence and indeed not infrequently multiple infarct dementia and senile Alzheimer's disease exist together. Both these conditions in life are only diagnosable by exclusion, since brain biopsy, although formerly practised in some circumstances, is clearly unethical at the present time and probably particularly so in the elderly. A form of senile dementia caused by diffuse Lewy bodies is also now being increasingly recognized.

Other conditions which must be considered as a potential cause of chronic intellectual impairment, and which should be excluded, are the subdural haematoma, neurosyphilis, parkinsonism, low-pressure hydrocephalus, drug side-effects, myxoedema, and B_{12} deficiency, as well as the other factors mentioned under the heading of the acute confusional state.

The investigations can usually be organized without hospital referral and should include:

(i) Biochemistry—urea and electrolytes, biochemical screen, especially liver function tests and bone biochemistry, and a plasma glucose.
(ii) Full blood count and ESR.
(iii) B_{12} and folate levels.
(iv) Thyroid function tests, i.e. T4/TSH.
(v) Syphilis serology.
(vi) Chest and skull X-rays.
(vii) MSU.
(viii) Other investigations indicated by the history of examination.

If a treatable cause is found then further action would depend upon the nature of the underlying condition. If, as can often be the case, one is no further forward in terms of discovering a potentially treatable lesion, the patient should be referred to the geriatric or psychogeriatric service if additional support is required, or there is a difficult behavioural problem to manage. In general, ambulant demented patients are probably best referred to the psychiatrist unless further investigations, e.g. a lumbar puncture and/ or an isotope or CT scan, are considered necessary.

Depression

Depression is more common in old age than is often realized, and is often difficult to diagnose but requires careful consideration, as in many cases treatment will bring about a beneficial improvement to an older person's life.

Treatment of depression usually involves prescribing medication but it is important not to forget that the supportive measures, such as relieving social isolation or loneliness, can be an essential part of the therapeutic approach . Although there are many drugs available to treat depression, some of which are claimed to be more appropriate for older people, it is important to use a drug with which one is familiar. The tetracyclic group appear to have fewer side-effects, particularly the anti-cholinergic problems, and, until recently, they were thought the best approach to adopt initially. However, the side-effect of blood dyscrasias (e.g. thrombocytopenia) have made it essential to monitor blood indices monthly during the first three months of treatment. So now many of us start with a tricyclic, initially in small doses. As in younger people, imipramine can be helpful in retarded depression and amitriptyline in those who are agitated. It is essential to remember that the elderly metabolize antidepressant drugs more slowly and they are particularly prone to the anti-cholinergic side-effects of these drugs, including a dry mouth, blurred vision, constipation, urine retention, tachycardia and postural hypo-tension, etc. Over-sedation is also a frequent problem. These problems appear to be least with the tricyclic agent lofepramine—and it is also safer in overdosage (Cassidy and Henry 1987). A suitable dose is 70 mg/12 h PO.

If an elderly person does not respond to a reasonable therapeutic trial, advice should be sought from a psychogeriatrician (if available). Although not generally used in elderly patients, it is sometimes necessary to consider monoamine oxidase inhibitors—the risk of hypertensive crises from dietary amines is traditionally emphasized in textbooks, but the risk has been greatly overstated: there have only been about 17 cases in 98 000 patient years (Bass 1989). These drugs may be particularly useful if there is overeating, oversleeping, marked fatigue, panic, hostility, phobias, or hypochondriasis. A suitable example from this group of drugs is phenelzine 15 mg/8 h PO. Avoid concurrent use with tricyclics, and MAOIs should not be started within 21 days of a dose of a tricyclic or related compound. Other risks include postural hypotension and the potentiation of other drugs (opiates, L-dopa, adrenalin, and related compounds often found in cough and cold remedies).

Flupenthixol 0.5–1.0 mg (in the morning as it may cause sleeplessness) is a helpful alternative to other agents—particularly if the patient has glaucoma (which is a contraindication to other antidepressants).

Other patients may need ECT if the more standard therapeutic approach is unsuccessful.

In all drug treatment of depression, remember six golden rules:

- Tell the patient over and over again that they are going to get better. Many elderly patients who are depressed have persistently negative thoughts: but once they believe that they can get better, many will, in fact, do so. Note: some elderly patients will never get better (in contradistinction to younger patients)—but we think it is justifiable to hide this fact from most patients, at least initially, because a positive approach from the doctor is itself such a valuable therapeutic asset.
- Explain to the patient that the drug will take some weeks to work.
- Explain that side-effects can become manifest before any therapeutic effect, and that the patient may well find him- or herself wishing to stop the drug at this stage. Warn the patient he may well feel this, but that he should persevere. Arrange to see the patient at two weeks to augment this advice.
- Explain that compliance is important. Consider asking the patient to bring his tablets with him (for counting) if compliance is likely to be a problem.
- Explain that treatment will need to be prolonged for some months after improvement to prevent relapse.
- Explain that treatment will need to be tailed off gradually.

Diabetes mellitus

Although many elderly people have a raised renal threshold for glucose, the upper limit of normal for the plasma glucose level is theoretically the same as in younger people. The increase in renal threshold will often allow them to run a plasma glucose level that is higher than normal without glucose 'spilling' into the urine and being detected there. This does not mean that the elevated glucose level is acceptable and any elevation in the plasma glucose must be considered pathological even if the raised renal threshold is protecting the patient from the effects of fluid and salt loss. A mild elevation of plasma glucose in the absence of glycosuria is acceptable, if there are no complications and the situation is carefully monitored.

A glucose level two hours after a meal is an effective screening test for diabetes mellitus in the elderly, and if the glucose level is greater than

10 mmol/l, this diagnosis is almost certain. It can be further confirmed by measuring a fasting glucose and detecting glycosuria in many patients. Reflectance meters have made it easier to undertake these measurements in the home. Although a glucose tolerance test is unnecessary in many elderly people, it is sometimes required in the instance of a difficult or borderline case. All glucose estimations should be performed on a blood sample which has been placed in a fluoride tube. It is not widely appreciated that red cell glycolysis may lower the sugar level by as much as half if left in an unfluoridated tube at room temperature for as little as three hours.

Many elderly diabetics do not need hospital referral, since the diagnosis can easily be made within the general practice setting. In a patient in whom the diagnosis has been confirmed, it is important to assess whether there are any complications, for example diabetic retinopathy or cataracts, peripheral vascular disease, coronary artery disease, or proteinuria indicating the possibility of diabetic nephropathy. The neuropathy of diabetes often seems to escape notice, possibly because the symptoms or signs are attributed to normal senescence. The traditional advice is that it should always be searched for and suspicion of its presence should be heightened in the presence of trophic lesions in the feet. However, it is interesting to note that in our own diabetic clinic, searching for neuropathy has been deleted from our check-list. We only have a fixed amount of time to spend with diabetic patients, and experience shows that it is more effective to spend the time with patients discussing diet and screening for retinopathy. The point is: *What do you do if you do find evidence of neuropathy? The answer is: Not much—except for trying to prevent deterioration by attaining normoglycaemia and stressing the need for patients to take great care of their feet, as they will not necessarily feel minor trauma*. And this means attention to diet: so why not attend to this matter at the outset? We used to feel guilty about deleting items on our check-list, commenting to ourselves that surely we should be striving for the best—and that this must include a systematic search for every complication. We now realize that this is not so—and that such a policy has serious side-effects. For us, these were that the doctor got irritated by the slowness of patients and their interjections, which prevented him from going down his check-list smoothly. We now realize that education is the single most important activity in our clinic and that *everything* else is secondary to this. This series of thoughts yields an interesting paradox: by agreeing to be second-rate (no 'full-house' of items on our check-list and adopting a relatively lax approach) we actually increase our effectiveness. We give our own check-list below, freely admitting that we do not fill in every item on every visit. Remember to advise chiropody.

Diabetes also causes an autonomic neuropathy in many people which is most usually evident as postural hypotension and bladder or bowel problems.

Before treating a patient for an elevated plasma glucose it is important to exclude other factors which may aggravate any hyperglycaemic tendency. These include drugs, especially some diuretics, corticosteroids, and perphenazine, in addition to other medical conditions, such as Cushing's disease, acromegaly, obesity, and thyrotoxicosis. With the exception of obesity and the drugs, the other conditions are of course rare. If one of these factors is discovered, appropriate treatment may well make it unnecessary to treat the plasma glucose itself.

The majority of elderly people with diabetes can be managed with a diet and an oral hypoglycaemic agent. Unfortunately, it is very difficult to encourage the elderly to lose weight, as food is so often one of the few pleasures left in their life. Sulphonylureas are usually the drugs of first choice, but it is probably best to avoid chlorpropamide, since this has a long half-life and is excreted by the kidney (it also causes alcohol-induced flushing). Renal impairment is commoner in the elderly, and also in the presence of diabetes and dangerous levels of chlorpropamide may build up in the circulation. Unless renal function is known to be normal it is probably best to use one of the shorter-acting sulphonylureas, e.g. tolbutamide (500 mg–1 g/12 h PO). These, however, stimulate insulin secretion, which may induce hunger and overeating and result in an increase in weight. If renal failure is present, the hepatically metabolized agents such as gliquidone are preferable. The dose of gliquidone is 15 mg (half a tablet) before breakfast initially, increased up to 60 mg/12 h PO. Sulphonylureas occasionally cause headaches. They are potentiated by azapropazone, co-trimoxazole and sulphinpyrazone. Concurrent use of sulphonylureas with nifedipine may impair glucose tolerance.

The problem of lactic acidosis associated with the prescription of biguanides is well known and is particularly likely to occur in patients with hepatic and renal impairment, especially in the presence of tissue anoxia, such as is associated with cardiogenic shock. Lactic acidosis hardly ever occurs in the absence of these factors, except with phenformin (which is why it has been discontinued). Metformin is now the only available biguanide. Its dose is 500 mg/8 h PO or 850 mg/12 h PO (both strengths of tablets are made). Other side-effects include anorexia (which may be an advantage) and decreased vitamin B_{12} absorption. Cimetidine increases its plasma concentration.

Insulin is needed in surprisingly few elderly diabetics, but when it is necessary to prescribe this, the principles of treatment are the same as in younger people. Failing eyesight and arthritic hands make it difficult for many an older person to administer their own insulin and it may well be necessary to train relatives or friends to administer it, or ask the district nurse to do it instead.

Any diabetic in whom control of the plasma glucose is difficult to achieve—and it must be remembered that hypoglycaemia is as dangerous as hyperglycaemia—or in whom there are complications is probably best referred to hospital for assessment, even though the subsequent management may well be left in the hands of the general practitioner.

Table 7.1 Proforma for a diabetic clinic co-operation card

Name:	Address:	Telepone:	DOB	
Treatment:				
Date of diagnosis:		Is a consultant actively involved?		
Date seen by GP	/ /	/ /	/ /	/ /	/ /
Glucose, mmol/l:				
(WORST values)				
pre-breakfast	...	...	...	...	...
pre-lunch	...	...	...	...	...
pre-tea	...	...	...	...	...
pre-bed	...	...	...	...	...
other times	...	...	...	...	...
Weight (kg)	...	...	...	...	...
BP (mmHg)	...	...	...	...	...
Right-eye: acuity	...	...	...	...	...
cataract	...	...	...	...	...
dot/blots	...	...	...	...	...
new vessels	...	...	...	...	...
other	...	...	...	...	...
Left-eye: acuity	...	...	...	...	...
cataract	...	...	...	...	...
dot/blots	...	...	...	...	...
new vessels	...	...	...	...	...
other	...	...	...	...	...
Pupils dilated?	...	...	...	...	...
Dark room used?	...	...	...	...	...
Retinal photography	...	...	...	...	...
Urine [Protein]	...	...	...	...	...
Diet advice	...	...	...	...	...
Feet	...	...	...	...	...

Ketonuria Ketonuria indicates diabetic keto-acidosis if glycosuria is also present, and should be treated appropriately. When an elderly patient presents with hyperglycaemia, the presence of ketonuria strongly suggests that diet alone will not be sufficient to achieve normoglycaemia in the long term.

Severe vomiting will also lead to ketonuria, but in the absence of glycosuria. In addition, starvation, or fasting such as occurs during enforced bed rest in a person living on their own, may also lead to ketonuria. Treatment of the underlying illness and appropriate support will usually remedy the situation.

Erythrocyte sedimentation rate

The erythrocyte sedimentation rate is often higher in older people than is consider normal in younger patients. Even a fall of 50 mm an hour has been accepted as normal by some authorities. At this level, however, careful consideration is necessary before dismissing it as a normal expression of ageing. It is not uncommon in older people to find an ESR up to or even above thirty mm per hour and this is where most of the difficulties of interpretation arise. This is especially true since there are so many other variables which affect the ESR, some of which are likely to be present in many of the elderly. These include the haemoglobin level itself and cardiac failure. In addition to this, technical factors also play a role in accelerating the rate of fall and perhaps one of the commonest of these is failing to ensure that the sedimentation tube is absolutely vertical. A deviation of a mere five degrees from the vertical can double the sedimentation rate.

If the elevated ESR is the only abnormal finding and the remainder of the laboratory investigations are normal and the history and examination unremarkable, it is not unreasonable to wait a short while and repeat it after a week or two. If the original value was spurious or due to a passing subclinical infection, it is likely that the result would be returned to normal. On the contrary, cryptic pathology previously present may have progressed to a point where it will declare itself on reassessment. Persistent elevation of the sedimentation rate requires further investigation.

If the ESR is very high, e.g. 100 or over, it is important to consider first the possibility of neoplastic disease, such as a neoplasm with secondary spread, a hypernephroma with or without secondaries, and also multiple myeloma, as well as non-malignant conditions, in particular the collagenoses. The history will indicate whether or not giant-cell arteritis and other related conditions, e.g. polymyalgia rheumatica, are a possibility. This can also cause the ESR to be very high. Appropriate investigations will indicate whether any of the other conditions mentioned are likely to be responsible.

The conditions mentioned above must also be considered if the ESR is elevated, but not as high as 100. In addition to the appropriate investigations for these conditions, it is also necessary to arrange for routine urea and electrolytes and biochemical screen, an MSU, a full blood count and film, and if appropriate sputum for culture and microscopy. GI tract pathology must also be excluded. Cryptic infection, such as tuberculosis and subacute bacterial endocarditis, is occasionally responsible and should be considered if no other cause is discovered. It is also important to remember that the elevated ESR associated with rheumatoid arthritis may persist for a long time after the joint disease has become extinguished, but one must not assume this to be responsible for an elevated ESR unless any other coexistent pathologies have been excluded.

Occasionally a low erythrocyte sedimentation rate is discovered in an older person. It does not usually present a problem and is more commonly associated with polycythaemia, hyperviscosity states caused by other diseases, and congestive cardiac failure.

The erythrocyte sedimentation rate is very non-specific and has little diagnostic significance. It is, however, helpful in alerting one that all is not well, and also when following the progress of a disease or its treatment.

Falls

Falls in the elderly should never be allowed to pass without consideration of their cause. It is easy to hear about an older person falling and just allow it to pass through one's mind without registering. However, the investigation of falls can often lead to worthwhile preventive medicine. It is very difficult to present a succinct account of the potential underlying conditions, since these are so legion (see Tinetti and Speechley 1989 for a full list). Instead, a practical approach is described which concentrates on the commoner causes, and those for which it is possible to take some action. In general, the history and examination are more helpful than investigations, which less frequently indicate a cause other than something which has been suspected already.

Although there is no substitute for a full history and examination system by system, there are four points of particular importance which should be sought during the history. These are as follows.

1. Vertigo

Many older people have great difficulty in accurately describing vertigo, giddiness, dizziness, etc. Falls are infrequently caused by true vertigo, but when this situation does arise it is important to exclude wax in the external auditory meatus before looking for more complex conditions, such as brainstem lesions and damage secondary to drug therapy. These will be responsible for only a few cases in older people, as also is Ménière's disease, a diagnosis with which many people are mislabelled.

An association between dizziness or giddiness and change in head position, e.g. extension such as when looking up to a high cupboard or lateral rotation as in looking both ways before crossing the road, indicates the possibility of cervical spondylosis and vertebrobasilar insufficiency.

2. Accident hazards

The commonest cause of falls is probably the accident hazard. Many minor falls of this nature are not reported to the doctor unless trauma ensues.

Common hazards include inadequate lighting, especially on staircases, loose mats, and trailing electric cables. These are common findings in the homes of the elderly.

3. Loss of consciousness

This is best confirmed from a reliable witness.

4. Relation to posture

Postural hypotension occurs more commonly than is generally realized and should be directly questioned for, and the blood pressure tested in the lying and erect positions in all people who have a history of falling. A drop in systolic pressure of 20 mm of mercury or more is usually significant, especially if associated with symptoms. The following underlying conditions need to be excluded: hypokalaemia, evidence of autonomic dysfunction and its possible causes, e.g. tabes and diabetes mellitus, and drug side-effects. Drugs that are particularly likely to be responsible include antidepressants, antiparkinsonian drugs, hypotensive agents, hypnotics, and diuretics. These can all aggravate or precipitate postural hypotension, which is then best treated by removing the cause. This should be followed where necessary by prescribing elastic stockings, but if it is difficult for the elderly person in question to put these on, stockinet of the tubigrip type may be very helpful. Finally, small doses of fludrocortisone may help in difficult cases (e.g. after consultation with a geriatrician). If after these measures there has been no improvement in the postural hypotension, further investigation is usually necessary and this is best carried out in a hospital outpatient setting.

One practical point of help is to counsel the patient to stand up or change his position slowly, and pause until the giddiness passes off. In many people this may obviate the need for elastic stockings or fludrocortisone.

The major systems will now be considered in turn:

(i) Cardiovascular system
If the falls are preceded or accompanied by palpitations, an ECG and in many cases a 24-hour ambulatory tape are necessary in order to exclude a dysrhythmia. Falls may also be a consequence of a Stokes–Adams attack, or an episode of bradycardia, and once again an ECG and a 24-hour tape are necessary in order to substantiate the diagnosis. Since both brady- and tachyarrhythmias may be symptomless apart from the falls, and often only occur sporadically, the standard ECG on its own is frequently unhelpful. For this reason any patient who has an unexplained history of falls should be considered a candidate for 24-hour monitoring unless this is inappropriate for other reasons.

(ii) Central nervous system

After excluding accident hazard, the majority of falls probably originate because of an abnormality somewhere in the central nervous system. Cervical spondylosis has already been mentioned, and a cervical collar may be helpful in some people. Unfortunately, degenerative arthritis in the neck is present in very many elderly people without any symptoms and is often an incidental finding in someone with a history of falling.

Disturbance of posterior-column function, in particular because of B_{12} deficiency or syphilis, will lead to impaired proprioception and a greater tendency to fall. Therefore, if joint-position sense is found to be defective, it is essential to estimate the serum B_{12} and perform syphilis serology. Occasionally, impaired joint-position sense is found to occur as part of a more generalized peripheral neuropathy, in which case it is important to exclude B_1 as well as B_{12} deficiency and diabetes mellitus, and also to consider the following conditions which occasionally occur in elderly patients as a cause of peripheral neuropathy—drugs and alcohol, lead poisoning (especially in older houses with lead pipes in soft-water districts), carcinomatosis, and amyloid.

More commonly than peripheral neuropathy, extrapyramidal symptoms, i.e. parkinsonian symptoms, are implicated. Before treating with antiparkinsonian drugs it is first necessary to ensure that the symptoms are not iatrogenic in nature. Phenothiazines, e.g. chlorpromazine and thioridazine are the commonest offenders and occasionally a butyrophenone, e.g. haloperidol, is responsible. Under these circumstances treatment is best initiated by withdrawing the offending drug. If it is not possible to do this for any reason, an anticholinergic/antiparkinsonian preparation should be prescribed, i.e. benzhexol or orphenadrine, rather than an L-dopa combination preparation. It is the rigidity and the bradykinesia which contribute most to falls, and these are probably best treated with an L-dopa preparation if the parkinsonism is not drug-induced. When prescribing these drugs one must bear in mind the possible side-effects that can occur.

Cerebellar ataxia most commonly results from cerebrovascular disease in older people and is occasionally responsible for, or contributes to, falling. Cerebellar dysfunction may also be produced by drugs, especially phenytoin, barbiturates, and alcohol, and occasionally by lesions in the cerebellopontine angle, e.g. an acoustic neuroma. A patient with cerebellar ataxia is best referred for further investigation, since occasionally a treatable cause is responsible, but it is worth withdrawing the drugs first if it is thought that these may be implicated.

Epilepsy also causes falls, and sometimes, if the seizures are not witnessed, the patient is found on the floor and the epileptic nature of the incident goes unrecognized. In old people living alone this can happen quite frequently without the diagnosis being considered. It is important to remember that epilepsy in older people may well be due to an old cerebrovascular accident scar, but can also result from space-occupying lesions and metabolic rather than physical causes. The onset of epilepsy in an older person should usually result in referral for further investigation and management.

There are other causes of falls due to abnormalities in the nervous system, and these include poor eyesight, e.g. owing to a cataract—extraction may well improve the situation—transient ischaemic attacks, and early dementia. The latter two are difficult to treat, but it is worth prescribing an aspirin tablet daily for someone with TIAs if there is not a contraindication and no other obvious cause for the attack.

(iii) Musculoskeletal system

Arthritis is the commonest cause of, or contributory factor to, falls as far as abnormalities of the musculoskeletal system are concerned. Osteoarthrosis, and occasionally rheumatoid arthritis with or without osteoarthrosis, are the types of arthritis that are most usually involved, but there are other conditions and it is important not to forget that diabetes and syphilis may be responsible for a grossly disorganized painless joint. An X-ray of the joint, especially if compared to the 'normal' side, will help establish the diagnosis. This is worthwhile since chronological age on its own is not a contraindication to standard surgical management and an accurate diagnosis is in any case necessary to justify medical treatment. However, falls are not really a reason, on their own, to recommend arthroplasty: pain is the best indication.

It is often forgotten that disease of the muscles themselves may contribute to a tendency to fall. Most commonly this takes the form of a proximal myopathy such as is found in thyrotoxicosis, Cushing's disease (which is rare in older patients), osteomalacia, electrolyte abnormalities, and carcinoma (especially of the bronchus). Any of these conditions, if considered, can be diagnosed with the usual laboratory or radiological investigatons, which can be arranged from the general practice setting. Occasionally, severe wasting of the quadriceps in a patient who has been in bed for a long time is difficult to differentiate from a proximal myopathy, but in the latter other muscle groups, including those of the upper limb girdle, are often also affected.

Just occasionally, a diabetic amyotrophy is responsible. This affects men more than women and is associated with wasting of the thigh muscles and severe pain.

(iv) Drugs

Falls are often iatrogenic, since many drugs may contribute to a tendency in this direction, especially if they affect the conscious level, e.g. hypnotics, sedatives, and antidepressants. Those causing postural hypotension have already been mentioned.

If the list of conditions described above can be excluded and the patient continues to fall, referral to a geriatrician is advisable.

The management of instability

Even after careful assessment and treatment many old people either continue to be at risk of falling, are afraid of falling, or both, and they and their relatives need help to cope at home. They need information about the factors which put their elderly relative at risk of falling, support and reassurance if they are very anxious, and involvement in the promotion of exercise and the use of walking aids, and preparation for a fall.

The promotion and exercise of confidence   The person who is afraid of falling may enter a vicious cycle.

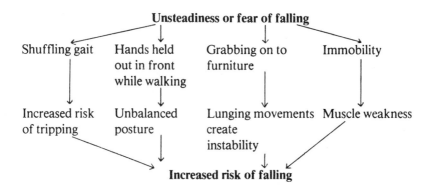

The promotion of exercises and the re-education of the patient are therefore of vital importance. The best approach is for a physiotherapist to pay a home visit to work with the old person and his relatives, but this is often difficult to arrange and visits to day hospital for physiotherapy have to be used as a basis for educating the patient and relatives.

The old person should be encouraged to: stand up straight; lift her feet and step out; walk slowly and steadily. There is also evidence that any form of exercise helps restore proprioceptive fitness: the promotion of exercise and confidence to go hand in hand. Encourage the patient to wear firm shoes with non-skid soles and ordinary (not high-heel) shoes. Point out the dangers of wearing slippers or bare stockings. If shoes are not worn because they are uncomfortable, is chiropody indicated?

Do what you can to reduce the risk of a fall. Does she really need her benzodiazepine or antihypertensive? Are her spectacles suitable? Is her environment suitable?

- Lighting (see Tinetti and Speechley 1988)
  Aim for absence of glare and shadows. Are the switches convenient? Try a night-light in the hall, bathroom, or bedroom.

- Floors
  Tack down carpet edges, have non-skid backing for rugs. Use non-skid wax on floors.
- Stairs
  Securely fastened, bilateral handrails. Do not store objects on stairs. Mark top and bottom of stairs with bright, contrasting sticky tape.
- Kitchen
  Fasten the table to the floor. Try to ensure that items are stored so that bending and reaching are not necessary.
- Bathroom
  Grab bars for baths, showers, and toilets. Non-skid mat in the shower. Use a shower chair and a hand-held shower. Raise the height of the toilet. Remove all locks so that emergency help can be given promptly.

The provision of walking aids (see p. 96)

Proper preparation for a fall   If it seems likely that the old person will fall, a number of measures can be suggested to minimize the risk of harmful consequences:

The old person should be taught how to rise from the ground. It is possible to teach people who are considerably disabled how to rise: for example the hemiplegic patient can be taught how to use his strong side to best advantage by a physiotherapist.

Arrangements should be made so that the person can call for help if he cannot rise, either by the provision of a telephone, or by asking neighbours to be prepared to notice a code or signal, such as three taps on the wall, or to call if the curtains are not opened. An alternative alarm system can be worn around the neck, signalling to a central point, so that help can be sent round at once. (Make sure that it is clearly stated who has a key, and note their telephone number.) Many Social Services departments provide finance and information to allow these alarms to be used.

By making all parts of the house as warm as possible the risk of hypothermia can be avoided.

Giant cell arteritis and polymyalgia rheumatica

Giant cell arteritis

Giant cell arteritis is a condition which rarely occurs in younger people and has a peak incidence after the age of 55 to 60. Together with polymyalgia rheumatica it is considered by many authorities to be part of a spectrum of disease with considerable potential morbidity in the elderly. The arteritis may affect arteries other than the temporal artery, and even extracranial vessels. It classically presents with a throbbing temporal headache associated with scalp tenderness noticed when brushing or combing the hair. It may also present with complications such as blindness and localized neurological signs. If the temporal arteries are affected they will be found to be thickened and tender and to exhibit reduced pulsation. The occipital arteries can also be felt in this way in some people in whom they are affected. The more local symptoms and signs are usually accompanied by constitutional disability with a fever and malaise.

Diagnosis

The diagnosis is supported by finding a high ESR, especially if it is elevated above 100, but can only be definitively confirmed with a temporal artery biopsy. Unfortunately this may be unhelpful, since occasionally there are skip lesions in the distribution of the arteritis and an apparently normal segment of artery may be excised. In addition it does not always affect the temporal arteries, as was mentioned previously.

Treatment

Treatment should never be delayed simply on the grounds of first obtaining a temporal artery biopsy or waiting for an ESR result to come back from the laboratory (it is cheap and easy to do your own ESRs in surgery—and this is perhaps the best solution). The risk of blindness or other occlusive arteritic event is sufficiently severe to warrant the immediate pre-scription of steroids, e.g. 40 to 60 mg of prednisolone daily. This is eventually reduced to the dose required to control the symptoms and main-tain the ESR at an acceptable level. Five to ten milligrams a day usually suf-fice and should be continued for one to two years and then cautiously withdrawn with close monitoring of the patient's symptoms and the ESR level. It must also be remembered that a recurrence may take the form not of giant cell arteritis, but of polymyalgia rheumatica. Any patient in whom giant cell arteritis is considered to be present should be referred to hospital as an emergency—if the general practitioner is not happy to start treatment himself at once.

Polymyalgia rheumatica

The major presenting feature of polymyalgia rheumatica is of pain and stiffness in the proximal limb muscles and the shoulder and pelvic girdles. This is usually worst in the mornings, and generalized constitutional upset including a pyrexia is usually present. It is accompanied by a high ESR and should be treated in the same way as giant cell arteritis. The symptoms usually respond dramatically to steroids, prescription of which is often a useful therapeutic test. Smaller doses of steroids, e.g. 20 mg of prednisolone daily, can be used initially if there is no evidence of an arteritis.

Hearing loss

As far as hearing is concerned, senescence and decay start almost from birth: perhaps this is the best illustration of the fallacy that there is, for humans, some golden age when we enjoy the full and simultaneous flowering of all our faculties, albeit briefly, before time confounds forever the gifts once so freely bestowed.

About 50 per cent of those over 80 years are deaf enough (i.e. a loss of ≥35 decibels) to get substantial improvement from a hearing-aid (the figure is 25 per cent for those 50–65, but only a quarter of these actually have aids fitted—even though they are free and anyway only cost the NHS £15–20 each). So it might well be worthwhile to screen for deafness using audiograms. Audiograms, however, need not be regarded as being essential to this task: simple clinical assessment is highly effective (Hickish 1989).

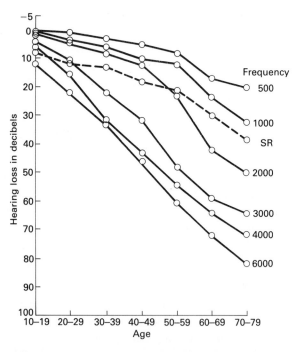

Fig. 7.1 Average audiograms (in males) for each decade of age from a large population survey (Gloring 1957).

The problem is not simply that as we get old we get harder of hearing: gerontologists have shown that there is an important interaction at work: the elderly cope less well with a predefined degree of deafness (Rabbitt 1988).

From a practical point of view, it is probably necessary to take seriously a person's complaint of deafness if they are having difficulty hearing normal conversations, and they can probably be definitively diagnosed as suffering from mild impairment if they are unable to interpret speech when a slightly louder voice than that employed in normal conversation is used.

The first step is to look in the ear and see whether there is a significant degree of wax in the external auditory meatus. If the deafness persists after this has been removed, testing with a tuning-fork will quickly indicate whether it has a conductive or sensorineural basis. If bone conduction (when the tuning-fork is placed on the mastoid process behind the ear) is better than air, then a conduction loss is present. Occasionally this is due to conditions such as otitis media and otosclerosis in the elderly, and the appropriate symptoms should be sought in the history. Unfortunately, sensorineural loss is commoner in older people and is rarely attributable to an underlying condition, and it is therefore not very often that one can treat a patient successfully. There is mixed opinion as to whether vascular disease on its own can lead to deafness of this type, but in theory it is possible. Other potential causes include drugs, especially streptomycin and quinine, and Ménière's disease. Again appropriate information to indicate these possibilities will be elicited from the history.

Help for the hard of hearing   The elderly person who is hard of hearing needs considerable help and encouragement. A number of aids and services are available to help people who are hard of hearing, and a check-list is given below:

(1)   Hearing aids, which should never be bought privately, except on the advice of the staff of the local NHS Hearing Aid Clinic.
(2)   Induction loop for television reception, allowing for the deaf person to receive amplified sound.
(3)   Flashing lights instead of the doorbell.
(4)   Ear-trumpets.
(5)   Telephone adaptations to allow the person to hear the phone ringing and conversation—leaflets and advice from the local telephone exchange.

However, these aids are only fully effective if the person is given support and help when using them. The best means of producing support and helping the person adapt to the loss of hearing is to introduce him to a club organized by the social worker for the deaf. In large towns and cities there are separate deaf and hard of hearing clubs, but in small towns it is more common for a single deaf and hard-of-hearing club to exist. These clubs are excellent rehabilitation centres and the deaf person can obtain all the information about aids and services in addition to advice on lip-reading and the maintenance of his aid. However, many people are reluctant to acknowledge that they are having increasing difficulty with hearing, and relatives need to be involved.

Advice for relatives   Relatives are as much in need of advice as deaf people. They need to be told not only about the range of aids and services available, but also how they can help the person who has difficulty with hearing. This advice can be summarized in a list of dos and dont's.

Do	Don't
Face the light (and be sure there is sufficient light, artificial if need be)	Mumble your words
Speak clearly and naturally	Exaggerate your lip movements
Sit or stand within two metres of your relative	Put your hand over your mouth when talking
Experiment until you find out how close you should sit or stand to make his hearing aid or lip-reading useful	
Look directly at your relative when speaking to him	Shout
Be friendly, casual, and tolerant	Smoke during your conversation
Have sympathetic understanding but not pity	Say one word over and over again, change the wording, and try again. Many words are difficult to see on the lips
Be patient with mistakes	Wear dark glasses. Much can be said by your eyes.
Watch for signs of fatigue	Allow the deaf person to become isolated: seek the advice of the social worker for the deaf if you feel he is becoming withdrawn
Write 'key' words on a pad (especially proper names) when necessary	
Encourage your relative to attend a club for the deaf or hard of hearing	
Encourage him to seek help if he finds his hearing-aid difficult to use or useless	

Deafness and mental health Deafness is associated with certain types of mental illness in old age:

- Anxiety.
- Depression.
- Paranoid delusions, sometimes with auditory hallucinations related to tinnitus.
- Confusion, due to sensory deprivation.

It is therefore essential to consider the contributions which deafness could be making when an elderly patient presents with one of these symptoms. Furthermore, clinical suspicion and questioning may not reveal a significant impairment in hearing. One study found that 60 per cent out of a sample of 253 people over the age of 70 had impaired hearing when assessed by pure-tone audiometry—which is twice the prevalence found by studies which relied on clinical asessment or self-reporting.

Hypercalcaemia

Many an elevated plasma calcium is factitious, being the result of stasis of the blood in the vein after a tourniquet has been applied. It is therefore necessary to repeat a calcium estimation on a fasting cuffless sample and also to correct the result in proportion to the serum albumin level. In the elderly two conditions in particular cause a rise in the plasma calcium. Probably the commonest is neoplasia, especially bronchial carcinoma, which can produce a parathormone-like substance, or carcinomatosis associated with multiple osteolytic deposits, and may be due to myeloma, a solid tumour, or a lymphoma. The second condition is hyperparathyroidism, but it occurs less frequently than the others. A neoplasm may often be suspected on the basis of the findings from the history and the examination in conjunction with a routine blood count, ESR, biochemical screen, and a chest X-ray. Where appropriate, other investigations are necessary, such as sputum cytology if a bronchial neoplasm is likely and an MSU to exclude the presence of red blood cells in the case of a hypernephroma. Other evidence indicating the presence of a neoplasm includes an elevated alkaline phosphatase, typical lesions on a skeletal X-ray, and multiple filling defects on a liver scan.

The presence of an elevated plasma calcium level with a decreased fasting plasma phosphate should lead one to consider the possibility of hyperpara-thyroidism. Additional evidence is also required before this diagnosis can be confirmed, the most important being of course estimating the serum parathormone level through the regional or supraregional assay service. It is, however, often helpful to undertake additional tests before estimating the parathormone level if this is difficult to obtain. An increased urinary calcium and phosphate excretion should also be found in a case of hyperparathyroidism, and a five-day course of corticosteroids will usually lower the calcium level in most conditions that cause hypercalcaemia, but not when it is due to hyperparathyroidism. Surgery is now undertaken more frequently for hyperparathyroidism in the elderly.

Other causes of hypercalcaemia include Paget's disease of the bone if the patient is bedridden or otherwise immobilized and less frequently vitamin D intoxication or a milk-alkali syndrome. These can usually be screened out on the basis of an adequate history, although it may be necessary to take this from a third person. There are of course other conditions causing hypercalcaemia such as sarcoid and thyrotoxicosis, but although they occur in the elderly they are an uncommon cause of hypercalcaemia.

A high plasma calcium is best treated in hospital.

Correction factor for plasma calcium level   If the albumin level is below 46 g/l add 0.025 mmol to the calcium level for every gram of albumin below 46 g/l. If above, subtract 0.025 mmol per gram of albumin above 46 g/l.

Hypertension

Research into the treatment of hypertension is yielding conflicting results— perhaps because there is no clear view on what counts as hypertension. One rule of thumb has been that the systolic BP is raised if it is greater than the patient's age plus 100. So a 75-year-old is 'allowed' to have a systolic BP of up to 175 mmHg. The trouble with this sort of rule is that it assumes that mortality and blood pressure are related—*whatever the age*. However, very confusingly, there is evidence of paradoxically increased survival (in men >75) with rising blood pressure (Langer, Ganiats *et al.* 1989)—and a less clear picture with women. Other studies have shown a slight reduction in stroke following treatment of hypertension in the elderly—but no effect on death from myocardial infarction. The conclusion from the recently published report from the European Working Party on High Blood Pressure in the Elderly is faultlessly worded but brilliantly opaque and character-istically unusable—to quote it in full: 'In patients taking active treatment total mortality was increased in the lowest of treated systolic or diastolic blood pressures. This increased mortality is not necessarily explained by an exaggerated reduction in pressure induced by drugs as for diastolic pressure a U-shaped relation also existed during treatment with placebo. In addition patients in the lowest thirds of systolic and diastolic pressures were characterized by decreases in body weight and haemoglobin concentration, and the patients in the lowest thirds of diastolic pressure taking active treatment also by an increased non-cardiovascular mortality, suggesting some deterioration in general health.'

Most studies have shown quite significant morbidity from antihypertensives. Furthermore, there is now very disturbing evidence that screening itself causes prolonged psychological distress—*even if the results are normal* (Stoate 1989). This may be from increased mortality-awareness and hypochondriasis. So what is the general practitioner to do? In our practice,* if we do stumble on a high blood pressure, we usually ignore it unless there is evidence of end-organ damage. We realize that this view depends on a somewhat selective view of the literature and that others may disagree strongly, including GKW especially if the blood pressure is very high—but in order to act consistently one has to be selective when elements in the literature are incompatible. We would be prepared to change our view if a safe hypotensive agent came on the market, and if screening was known to be an innocuous activity. In the mean time, we live by the aphorism *primum non nocere*.

Hypoalbuminaemia

Albumin levels are often a little lower in older than younger people without there being any pathological reason for this. When an old person becomes ill, however, the albumin often sinks to an even lower level, apparently because of the general debilitating effects of the illness. Despite this a low serum albumin can be caused by a specific condition and this must be considered before attributing hypoalbuminaemia to either age or a general effect of an illness.

The causes of a low albumin are legion, but as usual the history and examination may well be helpful. Amongst the commoner causes are malabsorption and an inadequate dietary intake, when supportive evidence will be found from a routine blood film and biochemistry, such as macrocytic or microcytic anaemia, or the biochemical concomitants of osteomalacia. If a gastrointestinal tract pathology is suspected from the patient's symptoms, amongst the commoner causes of a protein-losing gastroenteropathy are neoplasia, hypertrophic gastritis, Crohn's disease, and ulcerative colitis. Barium studies that can be arranged on an outpatient basis will often reveal the underlying pathology, but it may be necessary to refer the patient on to hospital for other procedures, such as endoscopy.

Liver disease is also a cause of a low serum albumin and if so there will often be other stigmata of hepatic pathology and derangement of the liver function tests. Protein loss from the renal tract will also lead to a degree of

* 'Our practice' means here, and in other places where the phrase is used, the practice of J. M. L. and partner in Ferring, West Sussex, England.

hypoalbuminaemia, especially if there is a nephrotic syndrome. In general, however, the minor degree of proteinuria found in the urine of many elderly people does not contribute significantly to a low serum albumin. Despite this proteinuria should be considered further in its own right.

Sometimes a low serum albumin is accompanied by a low serum sodium and urea and a low haematocrit, indicating the possibility of an expanded plasma volume, caused for example by secondary hyperaldosteronism. If this condition is suspected, it is probably best to refer the patient on to hospital for further investigation.

It is often extremely difficult to know when to investigate further a patient with a low serum albumin. There is a limit to the number of investigations that are reasonable in an older person, particularly when some of them are not going to reveal any treatable underlying pathology. In general, however, having excluded treatable conditions, it is reasonable not to investigate further a patient with a low albumin level unless it is very low (e.g. less than 25 g/l), continuing to fall, or associated with symptoms.

Treatment consists of correcting any underlying aetiological factor, since it is not possible to raise the serum albumin by alternative means such as an infusion of albumin. Symptoms may well have to be treated by simple measures, such as elastic stockings for peripheral oedema.

Hypocalcaemia

As mentioned above, a low serum calcium in an elderly patient may well be merely a reflection of the serum albumin level. It is therefore necessary to correct for the protein level and a formula is given on p. 86. If a low albumin is detected as the cause for hypocalcaemia, the hypoalbuminaemia should be investigated rather than the hypocalcaemia.

One of the most frequent causes of a low serum calcium in an older person is dietary vitamin D deficiency or malabsorption. Under these circumstances osteomalacia is often present and a low calcium will be accompanied by a low serum phosphate and an elevated alkaline phosphatase. This is indicated clinically from the history and additional investigations, since the findings on examination are rarely helpful. Amongst the tests that can be employed are the faecal fat estimation and barium studies. The latter will often define any underlying gastrointestinal cause for malabsorption if this is present.

Coeliac disease is not very common in the elderly but does occur, and if no other cause for malabsorption is found a jejunal biopsy may well be helpful. This would require hospital referral, although the other investigations mentioned up until this point can easily be arranged without sending the patient to hospital.

Chronic renal failure is often associated with resistance to vitamin D, and results in hypocalcaemia. There will usually be other evidence or a past history to indicate the existence of chronic renal failure. The serum alkaline phosphatase and phosphate levels, however, are often unhelpful and may be either normal or elevated.

Any patient who has undergone previous thyroid surgery must be suspected of having hypoparathyroidism if they present with a low calcium. This combination is uncommon but it is easily missed, since the scar is often almost invisible in an older person, and they may well have forgotten their previous thyroid surgery. Acute pancreatitis may also cause hypocalcaemia, but is not a common finding in the elderly. It is often associated also with glycosuria, and a plasma amylase level may confirm the diagnosis. This should be checked if a low calcium is accompanied by typical symptoms.

As usual one must always consider the drugs that a patient is taking when trying to elucidate the cause of hypocalcaemia. Amongst those most likely to be at fault are anticonvulsants and also carbenoxolone.

Hypokalaemia

The serum potassium level is not a good guide to the potassium balance of the body, since this element is found mainly inside the cells and the level in the blood will reflect partly the amount of water in the extracellular and vascular spaces. Potassium leaks out of cells when there is an acidosis, as occurs in renal failure and uncontrolled diabetes, and may produce a high level in the serum which does not reflect an increase in total body potassium. Indeed in the latter condition the body is often in negative potassium balance. Hypokalaemia, however, when accompanied by an alkalosis is always significant and may well be even in the absence of a high bicarbonate. Symptoms of a low potassium include a weak apathetic patient with a tendency to depression or confusion and lack of bowel motility resulting in constipation. Many general practitioners have the facilities to do an ECG, and in the presence of significant potassium depletion there will be flattening or inversion of the T waves with a prominent U wave and long Q–T interval.

The aetiology of a low body potassium is most conveniently considered in the following order, although each condition should be excluded since there is often more than one reason:

(1) **Diet** Illness and bed rest often lead to an inadequate diet because of an associated anorexia, or inability to prepare food. The potassium can quickly fall in these circumstances, and if the dietetic history indicates that the previous nutritional status was inadequate hypokalaemia will almost certainly have ensued as a result.

(2) **Drugs** There are several drugs which will lead to potassium loss. Diueretics are the chief offender. Amongst the other drugs that cause

hypokalaemia those most commonly encountered include carbenoxolone sodium and corticosteroids.

(3) **Loss of potassium from the gastrointestinal tract**   Both diarrhoea and vomiting can cause potassium loss if they are persistent. This is obviously apparent from the history and there will also be signs of dehydration, and an electrolyte estimation may well reveal the loss of other salts. Less common, but still an important cause of potassium loss from the bowel, is the patient with a history of purgative abuse. This tends to produce larger bulky stools with a high potassium content.

(4) **Loss of potassium into the urine**   The human kidney appears to have been developed to cope with that period of our evolution when we had a diet high in potassium and low in sodium. It is therefore very competent at conserving sodium and less so potassium. If supra-imposed upon this there is a degree of distal tubular dysfunction, as may occur in pyeloneprhitis and back pressure from an obstructive uropathy, the potassium-conserving ability of the nephron is seriously affected. If one suspects that the potassium is being lost in the urine, a 24-hour collection can easily be carried out in the patient's home and dispatched to the laboratory for estimation. It is probably best to send a complete collection rather than just an aliquot, if this is possible. The potassium excretion is not necessarily constant throughout the day. However, 24-hour specimens are notoriously unreliable. Even the best-motivated patients often forget to collect every time they micturate—and this may be compounded in the elderly bordering on confusion.

There are of course other causes for a low potassium, but these are less likely to be encountered, or noted in the patient's home environment. Examples are the treatment of a high blood glucose level with insulin, the administration of glucose parenterally, and the treatment of a severe anaemia, especially that due to B_{12} or folate deficiency.

The cause of the hypokalaemia is often obvious from the history, but if it remains obscure and the patient has obvious symptoms attributable to hypokalaemia, hospital referral is necessary to exclude the less common causes such as Cushing's syndrome, hyperaldosteronism, etc.

The treatment in the first place is correction if possible of the underlying cause. If potassium replacement is necessary it is best to use a preparation containing potassium chloride, since some of the other potassium salts exacerbate the hypochloraemia which often accompanies hypokalaemia. The upper gastrointestinal tract ulceration which is associated with potassium supplements is well known and is a good reason for avoiding tablets and prescribing instead a liquid preparation for the majority of elderly patients.

A severe hypokalaemia predisposes to cardiac dysrhythmias in addition to the other effects and is probably best treated in hospital with intravenous supplements.

Hyponatraemia

The serum sodium level in the fit elderly is the same as in younger people. However, many ill elderly people have a lower sodium than one would expect. In many instances no underlying cause for this is ever found and it rights itself as their condition improves.

One of the commonest remedial causes of hyponatraemia is probably sodium loss due to diuretic treatment. This should be suspected in anybody on diuretics, even if they still have significant peripheral oedema. There will often be other evidence of fluid and potassium loss in addition to the hyponatraemia. Under these circumstances, it is necessary to stop or reduce the dose of diuretic if this is possible.

Salt may also be lost from the kidneys as a result of salt-losing nephropathy, such as can occur in the presence of hydronephrosis, pyelonephritis, and possibly nephrosclerosis. This may well be accompanied by proteinuria and other evidence of renal impairment, such as an elevation of the urea and creatinine. In the majority of cases investigation should be limited to excluding remediable causes.

Salt loss from the gastrointestinal tract may occur in diarrhoea and vomiting and also in patients with intestinal obstruction or a paralytic ileus. These conditions are usually self-evident and appropriate treatment is along the standard lines. If the hyponatraemia is accompanied by hyperkalaemia, Addison's disease is a possibility, but this is extremely rare in the elderly. If Addison's disease is suspected, hospital referral is necessary.

Many elderly people have a low sodium as a result of a dilutional effect of water retention. This can occur for a variety of reasons, and possibly most commonly because of a defect in osmoregulation. It has been shown that even many fit elderly people have impaired osmoregulatory capacity. It may also be the result of other factors, for instance the inability of the kidney to excrete sufficient fluid because of poor renal blood flow, as may occur in conditions such as cardiac failure. Inappropriate secretion of antidiuretic hormone is another cause of dilutional hyponatraemia and is known to occur in a multitude of conditions, including malignancy, respiratory conditions including pneumonia and more chronic disorders, head injuries, and as a side-effect of some drug therapy, for instance chlorpropamide. This is best confirmed by measuring the osmolality of the urine, when it will be found that the hyponatraemia is associated with an inappropriately high urine osmolality and an elevated sodium content. Under normal circumstances hyponatraemia is associated with a very low urinary sodium as the kidney attempts to conserve the latter. The osmolality could probably be measured by the laboratory from a general practice setting, but if the diagnosis is confirmed, hospital referral for further investigation is probably best.

Hypothermia

This is defined as a central body temperature which has fallen to below 35 degrees centigrade. It is necessary to measure it with a low-reading rectal thermometer, or using a low-reading thermometer to measure the temperature of a freshly passed specimen of urine. It is a medical emergency and should lead to immediate hospital admission. The survival rate is low and death is precipitated by arrhythmias, and metabolic abnormalities, especially acidosis, hypoglycaemia, and hypokalaemia, among other causes. Prevention is as important as treatment, and the following factors should routinely be considered in every elderly patient before winter sets in:

1 **Exposure to a low environmental temperature**—e.g. an unheated and poorly insulated house. This unfortunately is the lot of many of our elders, and the grants which can be made available to assist in heating are insufficient, but a person at risk should be put in contact with the social worker so they can at least be considered for them.
2 **Pre-existing endocrinological abnormalities** Hypothyroidism and hypopituitarism lead to a fall in the metabolic rate and a greater than average chance of developing hypothermia. This should therefore be borne in mind in any patient who is known to suffer with either of these two hormonal abnormalities.
3 **Drugs** Various drugs can precipitate hypothermia either by causing body-heat loss by vasodilation and reducing shivering, or by causing sedation which results in exposure. Those sometimes implicated include chlorpromazine and other phenothiazines, barbiturates, antidepressants, and alcohol.

While awaiting ambulance transport (if admission is appropriate), it can be tempting to try and start the re-warming process. This can lead to complications, especially if it results in the body temperature rising at a rate of more than half a degree centigrade an hour. It is therefore best to wrap the patient well with blankets and employ heating to take the chill off the room, rather than at this stage to try and raise the patient's temperature artificially.

Some epidemiological figures are useful to bear in mind. In the UK in winter there are 40 000 excess deaths compared with the summer—most of these are in elderly patients, but very few of the deaths are due to hypothermia. It has been calculated that by each degree centigrade that the winter is colder than average there are about 8000 excess deaths. The Building Research Establishment has concluded that it is impossible to define a safe lower limit to house temperatures, but the risks incurred as the temperatures fall are summarized below (Lowry 1989).

21°C Room temperature recommended by the British Geriatrics Society.

18°C Parker Morris standard for living-rooms; comfort level for most people.

16°C Respiratory problems become more common.

13°C Parker Morris standard for kitchens.

12°C Cardiovascular changes increase the risk of myocardial infarction and stroke.

5°C Significant increase in the risk of hypothermia.

Social circumstances will often vitiate our attempts to make use of this information. Poor elderly people may not have much to do, and spend most of the day in sedentary postures, so they need more heat than younger, more active people. Poverty and cold go hand in hand with poor housing—i.e. just the sort of housing that is difficult to heat (ill-fitting doors and no insulation). This is underlined by the fact that elderly people spend a much higher proportion ($\times 2$) of their income on fuel than others. Central heating is the most efficient form of heating, but is an impossible luxury for many elderly people. Alternatives such as paraffin stoves are less efficient, create more water vapour, and are the source of many injuries. As an economy, an old person may choose to heat only one room. This encourages damp and condensation in the other rooms, and this may exacerbate health problems.

Immobility

Many patients are referred to a geriatrician with the diagnosis of 'The Gone off their Legs Syndrome'. In reality this is a very non-specific presentation of disease and underlying aetiological factors, which are often multiple, with one being the final precipitating factor, are so legion that it is only possible to give a few basic principles to consider.

1 **Generalized weakness**. This is a common complaint in patients presenting in this way, and although it is tempting to accept this as a non-specific symptom, it may indicate specific underlying abnormalities, including the myopathy of thyrotoxicosis, malignancy, osteomalacia, and other conditions such as polymyalgia rheumatica and not uncommonly electrolyte abnormalities. Although hypokalaemia is the commonest of the latter, hyponatraemia may also be a contributory factor.

2 **Arthritis**. Osteoarthrosis, and less commonly one of the other arthritic conditions, is commonly a contributory factor. The knees are most frequently involved, but the hip is also a site of predilection (see p. 58).

3 **Neurological conditions**. There are many potential neurological abnormalities which can result in or aggravate a tendency towards immobility. Probably the commonest include the unsuspected cerebrovascular

accident and parkinsonism. A clue to the former is the tendency of the patient always to fall, or be weakest on, one side. Parkinsonism is often drug-induced and should be suspected in anybody taking phenothiazines or haloperidol. Less commonly a peripheral neuropathy, such as that due to a neoplasm, B_{12} deficiency, or diabetes mellitus may be involved. The other neurological abnormalities are probably best sought for and investigated in a hospital setting.

4 **Cardiorespiratory abnormalities**. These are usually self-apparent from the symptoms, or examination of the patient, and include of course shortness of breath on exertion, chest pains, and intermittent claudication.

5 **Painful feet**. Pain in the feet is often tolerated by older people partly because they believe it to be inevitable, and partly because they know how difficult it is to obtain NHS chiropody. One common cause of foot problems is the difficulty which some old people have in cutting their toe-nails—in one study 18 per cent of men and 29 per cent of women could only cut their nails with help from others. Help is given either by their relatives or a chiropodist, and because relatives play such an important part in foot care they require simple instruction about the best means of cutting nails safely and how to choose a qualified chiropodist, if NHS chiropody is unavailable.

6 **Others**. Among the other conditions that must always be considered when old people are off their feet are the early stages of dementia, depression, timor cadendi (fear of falling) in which the cause of the falls is the most

---

Useful advice for elderly people and their relatives

Cutting toe-nails

- Do not cut the toe-nails of people with diabetes or vascular disease: seek expert advice.
- Always cut the toe-nail straight across; soaking the feet in hot water makes cutting easier.
- Press down the soft tissue on either side of the nail gently five times with a cotton tipped stick, after finishing the nail-trimming.
- If a nail is very thick and heavy rub a nail-file across the surface, keeping it flat and being careful not to file the skin.
- Seek the advice of a district nurse or qualified chiropodist if any part of the foot develops an ulcer, or has a cut which will not heal.
- Do not try to cut or pare corns with razor blades.
- If in doubt ask the advice of the district nurse or a qualified chiropodist.

Useful advice for old people and their relatives

Finding a chiropodist

If the National Health Service chiropodist cannot see an older person whose relatives cannot cope and they have to seek help privately, it is essential to choose a properly qualified chiropodist, that is one with the letters SRCh—State Registered or MChS—Member of the Chiropodial Society, after his name. Social benefits cannot pay the fees of private chiropody under any circumstances.

---

important factor to elucidate, minor foot pathologies which are more incapacitating than the doctor appreciates, and last, but not least, unsuspected fractures, especially of the femoral neck.

It can be seen that the majority of these conditions will be apparent after examining the patient and arranging appropriate investigations. Although the diagnosis can often be made at home, the majority of patients who have been off their feet for any length of time are probably best rehabilitated in a hospital setting because they need more intensive physiotherapy and occupational therapy than can be delivered at home, or through a Day Hospital or outpatient setting. It is probably best to refer a patient who has taken to his or her bed to a geriatrician, probably for a domiciliary visit, earlier rather than later in the course of their illness.

The management of immobility

Even after careful assessment and treatment of the causes of an old person's impairment of mobility, it is often impossible to restore mobility fully, and the old person and his relatives have to be given advice on how to cope with the immobility. A home visit by a physiotherapist, if it is possible to arrange this, or domiciliary occupational therapist, allows four possibilities to be explored:

• *Alteration of chair height*   Many old people are immobilized because the chair in which they sit is too low. This rarely causes complete immobility, but if mobility is to be encouraged it is essential to make it as easy as possible for the old person to stand up. The occupational therapist may:

Teach the old person how to stand up. Common mistakes are failure to move the bottom to the front of the chair and failure to position the feet correctly.

Use blocks under the feet of the chair.
Use a high 'geriatric chair'. These have arms, and the seat is 18 inches from the floor.

• *Advice on exercise*   If not given specific advice on exercise many people will assume that 'rest' is beneficial and will not take sufficient exercise. It is therefore important to give an 'exercise prescription', for example by saying that 'You can improve your health by walking to the back gate at least twice a day.' A physiotherapist may be able to help the elderly person and his family plan an exercise programme, setting goals which make successively greater demands on the person with the mobility problem.

• *The provision of mobility aids*   These should not be given too soon because they very quickly create dependence and can lead to a further loss of fitness: for example the 'Zimmer' walking frame can cause shoulder and spinal stiffness because of the forward lean it requires. Nevertheless mobility aids have a significant contribution to make and the needs of the patient for a mobility aid should always be considered. Possibilities are:

A walking frame.
Rails, either up the stairs or along the hall.
Rails at front and back steps or handles beside single steps.
Higher toilet seats, with grab rails nearby.
A wheelchair.

If blindness is the cause of the immobility the advice of the Mobility Officer for the Blind should be sought.

• *Adaptation of the dwelling*   The domiciliary occupational therapist can assess the need for:

A stair lift.
Ramps at the front or back door.
The installation of a downstairs toilet or bathroom.

Relatives should be advised never to undertake the expense of major alterations without the advice of the domiciliary occupational therapists.

Incontinence of faeces

This usually occurs for one of three major reasons:

1 Secondary to large bowel pathology, or diarrhoea from any cause.
2 Secondary to faecal impaction, when it is often associated with incontinence of urine as mentioned in the following section. This will not

always be apparent on rectal examination because the impaction can occur higher than the finger can feel, in which case, if it is suspected from palpating the descending colon, a plain abdominal film is necessary.

3 Secondary to neurological damage.

The presence of large-bowel disease or diarrhoea can usually be ascertained from the history and findings on examination. Whether or not further action is necessary depends upon the underlying pathology. If a local cause is discovered, however, appropriate treatment may be helpful, but in practice the response is often disappointing. Despite this, an attempt should be made, wherever feasible, to rectify an underlying condition.

Faecal impaction occasionally occurs as a result of bowel disease, and a sigmoidoscopy and barium enema may be necessary, either before or after clearance of the rectum depending upon the practicalities of the situation. A single enema or suppository is extremely unlikely to adequately clear the rectum and descending colon of retained faecal residues. It is necessary to continue to administer intermittent enemas until the rectum can be seen and felt to be clear and the descending colon is found to be free of faecal residues on palpation. Occasionally, a plain abdominal film is necessary to confirm this. Having cleared the impaction, the next step is to maintain this state of affairs by keeping the patient's bowel habit regular with the aid of a dietary fibre or mild laxative regime. Aggravating factors, such as codeine-containing analgesics, should also be avoided. Additional fibre in the diet is probably best tried initially, in order to avoid the need for laxatives if possible.

Neurological damage can lead to faecal incontinence in a variety of ways, but the commonest is that occurring in a confused or demented patient. If the latter is responsible, it will usually be discovered that the patient is passing formed motions rather than the semi-liquid material typical of faecal soiling due to impaction. It is necessary to remember, however, that faecal impaction can occur, and frequently does, in demented patients. If a treatable cause has not been discovered, faecal incontinence is often best treated by using a

---

Useful advice for patients and their relatives

The prevention of constipation

The daily use of laxatives should be discouraged, although it can be difficult to break a habit which has lasted for decades. An increase in fibre intake should be suggested instead, but they should be told to start with a small amount of bran, or one slice of wholemeal bread for example, and then increase the amount. A large helping of Allbran® or bran can cause colic and explosive bowel actions in some people.

constipating drug, e.g. codeine phosphate, and arranging for an artificial bowel evacuation twice weekly with the help of suppositories or an enema. Particular care must be taken with this regime to avoid faecal impaction!

Incontinence of urine

The diagnosis and management of incontinence of urine is often a perplexing problem, with so many theoretical aspects that on occasions it is difficult to know where to start. In the elderly it is best to adopt a practical step-by-step approach, and the following is a suggested sequence of diagnostic and management steps.

1. *Exclude apparent incontinence*

By this is meant those circumstances where a patient is, in common parlance, 'caught short'. In reality they do have control of micturition to some extent, but for some reason they are unable to get to the toilet or their bottle quickly enough. Probably one of the commonest examples is the urgency or frequency associated with infection in the lower urinary tract, and not infrequently it may also be the result of urgency caused by a potent diuretic. The loop diuretics, i.e. frusemide and bumetanide, are the commonest causes of the latter. A careful history and examination of a midstream specimen of urine will help indicate whether one of these factors is responsible, or as is occasionally the case, a contributory factor.

Another circumstance in which apparent incontinence arises is the bedbound patient who uses the bottle, but who manages to spill some of the urine after he has passed it. If this happens at night, the patient's memory of the events occurring in the preceding hours may be somewhat hazy, and often they are not certain how they managed to become wet.

Although there are many other situations which may lead to apparent incontinence, there is one other situation which particularly merits attention, and this is the patient who finds himself in unfamiliar surroundings. It is not unusual for a person to become incontinent shortly after admission to an old persons' home for example, when they were previously continent. This is not just caused by the personal upset at being in a different environment, but probably also in many cases because they are unable to orientate themselves and find the toilet quickly enough, or because the toilet is considerably further away from their own room or the day room than it was from their living-room or bed at home. In these circumstances it may take a while for the patient to adjust, and if this process is proving traumatic, a bedside commode or bottle may well overcome the difficulties as far as nocturnal incontinence is concerned. A careful history and an awareness of the different environment into which a patient has moved may well lead to greater understanding

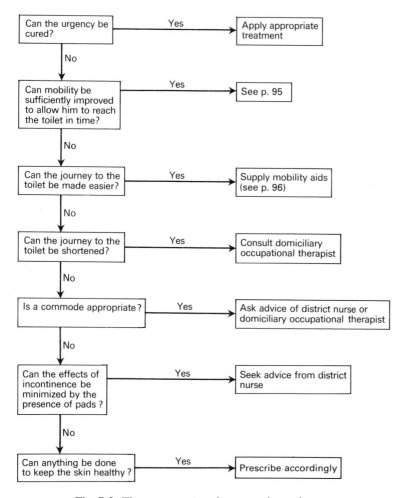

Fig. 7.2 The management of apparent incontinence.

of this problem when it arises. A flow-diagram of the management of apparent incontinence is shown in Fig. 7.2.

2. *Retention with overflow*

This should be excluded next, and it is usually not difficult to diagnose. A full bladder can be felt bimanually or percussed, and pressure over the lower abdomen will often lead to the patient experiencing a feeling of the need to micturate. If necessary, a plain abdominal X-ray will show a large soft-tissue mass arising out of the pelvis. If retention of urine is confirmed the first step is to exclude faecal impaction as its cause, and although this is also frequently associated with faecal soiling, this is not always so. The treatment of faecal impaction is considered on page 97. Another common cause of retention with overflow is the prescription of anticholinergic drugs, especially tricyclic antidepressants and antiparkinsonian treatment. Retention with overflow after the prescription of any of these drugs may act on its own or aggravate a pre-existing condition. The first step therefore is to exclude faecal impaction and review the patient's drugs, and this is usually simple and does not require hospital referral.

The next commonest cause is probably prostatic hypertrophy if the patient is male, in which case he should be referred to a urologist for further consideration. It is not correct to assume that a patient is too old for surgery, and a TURP especially is a relatively safe and simple procedure even in the disabled. In some patients where this is not appropriate, a catheter draining into a discretely placed thigh collecting-bag may well be the long-term solution to their problems.

In theory, there are many other causes for retention with overflow, but in the elderly they are less common than those mentioned above. Occasionally, an atonic neurogenic bladder occurs as a complication of diabetic neuropathy or tabes, when the history and other evidence of autonomic dysfunction or syphilis may indicate such a possibility. In general, however, these diagnoses are best left to the urologist and it is probable that in any patient in whom incontinence is associated with retention of urine, referral for a further opinion is mandatory.

On the practical side, if it is decided to empty a large distended bladder, it must be remembered that this should be done slowly to avoid the risk of intravesical haemorrhage from delicate vesical veins.

3. *Stress incontinence and senile vaginitis*

There are two conditions that are particularly important in women and merit consideration next. The first of these is stress incontinence, which often dates back to pelvic-floor damage occuring during childbirth, and which may also be associated with a prolapse. The nature of this type of incontinence is usually apparent from the history and examination, and usually requires referral to a gynaecological clinic, although it is often worth trying a ring pessary first.

Senile vaginitis is associated with incontinence because some of the urethral tissue and the trigone at the base of the bladder have the same embryological origin as the vagina. A local oestrogen preparation, as well as treating the vaginitis, will also often remedy the incontinence. Occasionally oral hormone preparations are necessary, but these are associated with more severe side-effects. Whichever regime is adopted, intermittent courses are required, the interval between being gauged in each particular patient on a trial-and-error basis.

4. *Mental impairment*

Incontinence is often associated with intellectual impairment, whether this is the result of an acute confusional state or part of an existing dementia. When associated with an acute confusional state this is usually obvious, and attention to and remedy of the underlying disorder is associated with a return of continence. In more chronic mental impairment, however, the situation is more difficult to resolve and often responds best to regular bladder-emptying in conjunction with an incontinence chart, recording frequency and time of the episodes of incontinence. This may help indicate the most appropriate times to toilet a patient, and sometimes results in the establishment of a regular pattern.

It is also important to remember that sedative drugs, both those prescribed for use during the daytime and at night, may also lead to incontinence because of a diminished awareness of the need to void urine. This is most commonly a problem at night when associated with the prescription of hypnotics. In the latter circumstance, discontinuation of drug or replacement with a short-acting preparation which promotes sleep but does not continue to impair the conscious level may well help rectify the problem.

5. *The uninhibited neurogenic bladder*

This is unfortunately the situation in many elderly patients, and is often irremediable. Lesions involving the frontal cortex are commonly involved, but damage to the other parts of the cerebrum may also be responsible. The patient is unable to prevent spontaneous bladder contractions, such as those that inform us that our bladder is full and which we constantly override until such time as it is convenient to pass urine. A cystometrogram is required to diagnose this with certainty, and geriatric referral is usually indicated to enable this to be arranged. Some pharmacological agents are occasionally helpful, and it is often worth trying preparations such as terodiline and/or flavoxate before resorting to other measures. They need to be taken at an appropriate time in relation to the incontinence, and a chart is usually helpful in this respect. Finally, it must be remembered that they have side-effects and also should not be used in patients with glaucoma. These agents should not be used in the presence of obstruction. This can be diagnosed by asking the patient to empty the bladder completely. Then pass a catheter and measure the residual volume. A residue of less than 50 ml rules out obstruction, and it is then possible to try drugs—without the need for a cystogram.

6. *Psychological urinary incontinence*

Some elderly people are incontinent for psychological reasons of which they are not fully aware. Common examples are:

- Punishment incontinence—usually to punish relatives.
- Attention-seeking incontinence. Consider how much attention someone in an old people's home receives if he is incontinent, compared with the amount he receives if he takes himself to the toilet in time.
- Avoidance incontinence—for example to avoid admission to an old people's home.

It is uncommon for psychological factors to be the sole cause of the incontinence, but they often complicate the problem and influence the severity of it.

Unfortunately, in many patients the incontinence has a multifactorial basis and diagnosis and treatment of one contributory pathology does not always lead to the restitution of continence. On the other hand, incontinence is such a disabling impediment both physically and socially that it is well worth systematically going through all the steps in every incontinent patient.

The management of incontinence

After diagnosis of the cause and treatment, if treatment is possible, the management of incontinence has to be planned with the old person and his relatives.

Objectives of management:

1 To protect the dignity of the patient.
2 To protect the skin of the patient.
3 To save the old person, his relatives and helpers from unnecessary work.

The advice of the district nurse is of central importance to the family in achieving these objectives, but referral to hospital may be useful, particularly if the hospital has a specialist incontinence advice service, usually a nurse or physiotherapist, who can try out the full range of aids and appliances. The many aids which are available can be arranged in order of acceptability and effectiveness in preventing damage to the skin. The most acceptable should be tried first.

Incontinence aids in order of acceptability:

1 Urinals are very useful for people whose main problem is reduced mobility.
2 Plastic pants with absorbent pads. A wide range of these are now available.

3 Catheterization. In those patients in whom no treatable cause for the problem is found, the choice of long-term solution is limited. A catheter draining into a discreetly placed thigh collecting-bag attached to a waistband is probably the most satisfactory long-term solution for many people.

Nocturnal incontinence Relatives need information about the prevention of incontinence at night. Firstly they should be told that limitation of fluid in the evening is not always effective and that it can cause problems. Secondly, the need for a commode or urinal in the bedroom should be discussed, even when the old person is able to reach the toilet during the day.

The risk of falls at night due to a combination of postural hypotension and peripheral vasodilation can be prevented by leaving a landing light on, and the provision of a commode or urinal.

If nocturnal incontinence is a problem, medication should be reviewed. The half-life of many tranquillizers is increased in old age, and even if the old person is not receiving a hypnotic, the effects of his daytime medication may be contributing to his noctural incontinence. If he is receiving a hypnotic this can be withdrawn with the substitution of a more active daily programme and a settled evening activity-pattern to establish pre-sleep ritual.

Nocturnal incontinence check-list

- Is medication a contributory factor?
- Would a commode or urinal help?
- Does the old person have enough light to see what he is doing?
- Have the relatives or the home-help been advised on the best way to make up the person's bed? Again, the advice of the district nurse is of vital importance.

Incontinence counselling

Although mentioned last it is of primary importance to take into account the emotional aspects of incontinence from the moment of presentation. Incontinence gives rise to feelings of disgust, fear, shame, humiliation, and depression, which may be followed by apathy and hopelessness. For the relatives it can be a source of frustration and anger, 'the last straw'. It is therefore essential that the affected person and his relatives be given the time and the encouragement to discuss their feelings about one of the most feared problems of old age.

Incontinence check-list

- Is the problem really incontinence with complete loss of control, or is it 'apparent incontinence' due to a combination of urgency and immobility?

- When apparent incontinence has been excluded, a five-step assessment is indicated:

Step	Possible cause	Test
1	Retention with overflow —faecal impaction —prostatic hypertrophy	Rectal examination
2	Stress incontinence or senile vaginitis	Vaginal examination at least or inspection while patient performs cough test
3	Mental impairment	Perform simple mental assessment. Review drugs and exclude alcohol abuse
4	Psychological factors	Review social significance of incontinence
5	'Neurogenic bladder'	Referral for full assessment with cystometrogram

---

Useful advice for old people and their relatives

Controlling the smell

- Soak soiled or wet clothes or linen as soon as possible.
- Dispose of incontinent pads by wrapping them in newspaper or putting them in plastic bags as soon as possible. Then put the 'parcel' in a larger plastic bag.
- Try *Nilodar®*, which is a neutralizing deodorant to combat smells. It actually neutralizes smells, and needs only a few drops in the commode or pad. It is available from most pharmacists.
- Try to keep the house and room well ventilated.
- Remember that the old person may not detect the smell if he never leaves it.

Useful advice for old people and their relatives

Coping with laundry

The two main difficulties are smell and staining. Both get worse when bedding is exposed to air. Wet or soiled clothing or bed-linen should be removed as soon as possible and soaked in cold water in a covered bucket. *Napisan*® should be added to the water, and the clothing can then be washed in the usual way.

Biological powders are not necessary if soiled clothes and sheets are soaked quickly.

Enquire about the possibility of help with laundry from the Incontinence Laundry Service

---

Jaundice

Jaundice is investigated along similar lines to those used in younger patients, but the results may be more difficult to interpret, as other diseases may also be reflected in the biochemical findings, e.g. bone disease causing an elevation of the alkaline phosphatase. If it is difficult to estimate the different isoenzymes of alkaline phosphatase it is usual to check a 5-nucleotidase level whenever there is any doubt, since this is only raised when there is liver disease and is unaffected by conditions of bone. The history and examination are often revealing when determining the most likely cause for a patient's jaundice: for instance, signs of chronic liver disease indicate long-standing hepatic damage rather than a more acute episode, such as a stone blocking the common bile-duct. The normal range of bilirubin level should be taken as the same in older patients as in younger people.

Jaundice is most conveniently divided into the usual three major types, i.e. obstructive jaundice and hepatocellular jaundice and the less common haemolytic jaundice.

Obstructive jaundice

Obstructive jaundice is probably the commonest form of jaundice in the elderly and is characterized by finding an elevated alkaline phosphatase. Although the transaminases are also usually raised, relatively speaking this is to a lesser degree than the alkaline phosphatase. Although rarely tested for there will also be the usual findings in the urine (see p. 108) in conjunction with the history of dark urine and pale stools. It is not uncommon for a gallstone to produce a severe jaundice and yet itself be painless, even though the old adage that painless obstructive jaundice is due to a neoplasm is very often true—particularly if the gall-bladder is palpable (Courvoisier's 'law').

Among the commonest neoplasms are those of the head of the pancreas, the stomach, multiple secondaries from other sites, and more rarely a carcinoma of the biliary tract itself. If a more diffuse condition, such as a lymphoma, is responsible there will usually be splenic enlargement and possibly lymphadenopathy.

Drugs do not cause jaundice in the elderly as frequently as they once did, since phenothiazines, especially chlorpromazine, are not prescribed as often as they once were. Nevertheless, they should be considered as a potential cause. A quick look at the patient's drug history may well fail to disclose the culprit—it is all too easy to forget to record a single dose—e.g. of pro-chlorperazine which may have accompanied an opiate injection for example. As well as phenothiazines, sulphonylureas and erythromycin are amongst the drugs that can be responsible.

Most patients with obstructive jaundice should be admitted to hospital, but if the jaundice is not severe and the patient is well enough, it may be possible to arrange further investigations as an outpatient. Occasionally a plain abdominal film will reveal gallstones. The majority of these, however, are radiolucent and even when found are not necessarily responsible for the jaundice. Particularly helpful is an ultrasound scan, and it is sometimes possible to arrange for one of these to be performed urgently to confirm the diagnosis. This can be a help in deciding whether or not the patient should be admitted to hospital, and will also show secondary deposits if present, allowing some patients the possibility of terminal care at home. An oral cholecystogram is unhelpful if the patient is clinically jaundiced, but intravenous cholangiography may reveal useful information if the bilirubin level is less than 33 μmol/1 (2 mg per 100 ml). Sometimes barium contrast studies are appropriate and may show the presence of an upper GI tract tumour.

Hepatocellular jaundice

In hepatocellular jaundice the SGOT and LDH levels rise, relatively speaking, to a higher level than the alkaline phosphatase. The urinary abnormalities are described below. The commonest cause of hepatocellular jaundice in the elderly is probably alcoholic cirrhosis (which frequently has an obstructive component to it). This may well be suspected from the history, although alcoholics are extremely adept at minimizing or denying their alcohol intake; but there will usually be evidence of long-standing liver disease on physical examination, including signs of portal hypertension. A barium swallow will often show the presence of oesophageal varices.

More 'pure' causes of hepatocellular jaundice include viral hepatitis, chronic active hepatitis, and drugs (halothane, paracetamol, methyldopa, and barbiturates).

Haemolytic jaundice

This is an uncommon finding in older people and is most easily confirmed in the general practice setting by testing the urine (see p. 108). A mild degree of haemolysis, however, may be present in untreated pernicious anaemia because of the shortened life-span of the macrocytic red cells. Other causes of haemolysis which should be suspected in the elderly include a severe infection, usually with septicaemia, and pulmonary infarction in a patient who has congestive cardiac failure. It can also be caused by certain drugs, and among those that should be suspected are methyldopa, mefenamic acid, penicillin, phenacetin, and salicylates.

Old people rarely suffer with hereditary spherocytosis and paroxysmal nocturnal haemoglobinuria, but idiopathic autoimmune haemolytic anaemias may occur at any age and may be associated with warm or cold antibodies. The cold antibody variety is more prevalent in the elderly and is often associated with Raynaud's phenomenon and haemoglobinuria in addition to the anaemia. A positive direct Coombs' test and an excess of cold antibodies in the serum confirm the diagnosis.

Other causes of haemolytic anaemia in the elderly include the secondary autoimmune disorders, which are often associated with other underlying conditions, in particular lymphomas, paraproteinaemias, and collagenoses. A patient with a haemolytic anaemia is probably best admitted to hospital, although the treatment of the anaemia itself may be relatively simple if it is due to one of the warm antibody types, since steroids are often helpful, as may be immunosuppressive therapy, although it may be necessary to resort to splenectomy in some cases. These measures are occasionally beneficial in the cold antibody types, but they are more difficult to treat.

Enzyme abnormalities

Alkaline phosphatase   Although the normal range for alkaline phosphatase levels is probably the same in older as in younger patients, we frequently ignore minor elevations. The two most important sources for this enzyme are liver and bone. Most of the hepatic alkaline phosphatase is concentrated in the epithelium of the bile-ducts, which probably explains the high levels obtained in an obstructive process. The highest levels of alkaline phosphatase may be associated with a tumour of the biliary duct epithelium, although this is uncommon.

Osteolytic abnormalities of bone require an accompanying osteoblastic reaction for there to be an elevation of the alkaline phosphatase. Most commonly this is associated with secondary bone tumours, in particular from the breast and prostate. Occasionally, it also happens in multiple myeloma. In all of these conditions, however, the alkaline phosphatase may also be elevated because of hepatic involvement. Two other bony causes of an elevated alkaline phosphatase are Paget's disease and the presence of a healing fracture.

A routine biochemical screen usually includes liver-function tests and bone biochemistry and will therefore in the majority of cases help to differentiate between a hepatic and a bony cause for the elevated alkaline phosphatase level. If, however, the calcium, phosphate, and liver-function tests are normal, it may be necessary to estimate the iso-enzymes or the 5-nucleotidase level. This is an enzyme that is specific to liver disease and indicates that the alkaline phosphatase is raised because of hepatic impairment, although occasionally there may be coincidental bone involvement, e.g. with secondary deposits in both sites.

Lactate dehydogenase (LDH)   An elevated LDH may be an accompaniment of many conditions. Most commonly it indicates hepatic impairment or a recent myocardial infarction. In the latter case there is the typical pattern of a peak approximately two to three days after the infarction has occurred. It may also rise in pulmonary infarction, in association with a megaloblastic anaemia, and occasionally in a patient with a cerebrovascular accident. The underlying aetiology can be ascertained with the help of a biochemical screen, a blood count, and an ECG.

Aspartate transaminase (SGOT)   This is usually elevated in liver disease, and high levels are a marker of hepatocellular pathology, since the rise in obstructive jaundice is usually moderate. It also rises after a myocardial infarction, with peak values a little in advance of the peak in the LDH level.

Biliary pigments in the urine (Table 7.2.)

Bilirubin   Bilirubin in the urine indicates the presence of obstructive jaundice. The obstruction to the outflow of bile results in spill-over into the

Table 7.2 Biliary pigments in the urine

	Bilirubin	Urobilinogen
Normal	None	Small amount
Prehepatic jaundice (e.g. haemolysis)	None	Increased
Hepatocellular jaundice	Present	May be increased then absent, depending on cause
Posthepatic jaundice	Present	Absent

blood of some conjugated bilirubin which is secreted in the urine, and conversely, the absence of bile in the bowel produces the pale stools and loss of urobilinogen from the urine. The presence of the latter relies upon the absorption from the bowel and excretion by the kidney.

Urobilinogen   Urobilinogen in excess of the urine is usually a consequence of a haemolytic process. A haemolytic anaemia is best confirmed with the aid of a blood count and film, and a Coombs' test, which will be positive in the majority of the autoimmune haemolytic anaemias. Initially these should be considered to be drug-induced until proved otherwise, as described above. Occasionally, a haemolytic process can be complicated by an obstructive element owing to the formation of pigment gallstones, and this situation may be difficult to unravel.

Treatment   Unless the cause of the jaundice is immediately apparent and does not require onward referral, or the disease is static, most jaundiced patients should probably be referred to hospital. It is particularly important to exclude remediable conditions and those that can be ameliorated. Examples of these include the silent stone and the bypass procedures in somebody with malignancy at the head of the pancreas. In the former case, the patient can look forward to a normal life-span after a successful operation, and in the latter often several months of symptom-free life until terminal care is required.

Leg ulcers

There are many potential causes of leg ulcers, varying from the commonly encountered arterial insufficiency and ulceration associated with varicose veins, to less common conditions such as those associated with severe ulcerative colitis and the haemolytic anaemias. It is important to try and establish the cause wherever possible, since the treatment for one condition may aggravate another if the diagnosis is in error, e.g. elevation of the legs for stasis ulceration in a patient with vascular insufficiency. There may be indications in the history which will lead one to suspect the presence of a particular type of ulceration, for instance diabetes mellitus indicating the possibility of peripheral vascular disease.

Varicose ulcers can usually be suspected from their characteristic site, the associated pigmentation, and the history of varicose veins. The presence of oedema may also be a helpful factor in arriving at the diagnosis, but it is more difficult to interpret, since there are so many causes of ankle swelling in the elderly. Varicose ulcers are best treated by rest with the legs elevated. Elevating the foot of the bed at night in a patient with no contraindication (e.g. orthopnoea, hiatus hernia, or peripheral vascular disease) will also help speed healing.

Ulcers resulting from peripheral vascular disease are the most difficult to heal. Often all one can do is combine an attempt to promote healing with measures to treat the underlying predisposition, if any, to vascular disease in the hope of slowing down a tendency to ulceration in the future.

In diabetes mellitus the skin may break down not just because of vascular insufficiency, but also because of the neurological sequelae of this condition, which results in impaired awareness of local trauma.

Any patients in whom there is ankle oedema and who sustains minor trauma is a candidate for a wound that will be slow to heal. It is as important to treat the underlying oedema as the wound itself, and this will require *Tubigrip*® type stocking rather than diuretic therapy, unless the oedema is caused by cardiac failure.

In bedbound patients pressure sores are also a cause of leg ulceration, but these are discussed elsewhere (p. 121).

The initial treatment of a leg ulcer consists in looking for and remedying where possible any underlying cause, as mentioned earlier, cleaning the ulcer, and applying simple dressings. Half-strength eusol should be avoided by using instead saline or one of the modern antiseptic solutions. Chronic leg ulcers often support a variety of bacteria, whose importance is a matter of controversy. If there is evidence of surrounding cellulitis to a significant extent, systemic antibiotic therapy rather than topical application is indicated. Topical antibiotics may do more harm than good and often precipitate contact dermatitis, with an aggravation of the ulceration. It is considered by some authorities that anaerobic organisms, especially streptococci and *Bacteroides* species, may play a more significant role than formerly recognized. A seven-day course of metronidazole (e.g. 400 mg/8 h PO) may speed healing if an anaerobic infection is discovered.

A patient's nutritional state may also be important in promoting healing, and if there is any cause to suspect malnutrition, attention should be paid to the patient's diet and the possible need for vitamin replacement.

Recalcitrant leg ulcers are probably best referred to hospital for further consideration, which may involve skin biopsy and/or the possibility of grafting in appropriate cases, although many ulcers will heal with a spell of bed-rest and intensive nursing support. Pinch skin grafts may be performed successfully in general practice, as follows. After local anaesthesia, pieces of skin (0.2–0.5 cm across) on the anterior thigh are raised on a syringe needle and detached using a scalpel. They are then transferred to the ulcer and covered with a non-absorbent dressing.

Malabsorption

Malabsorption is indicated by finding a similar biochemical and haematological picture to that described under the heading of malnutrition (see below). The absence of steatorrhoea does not exclude this condition, and many elderly people have significant malabsorption without any evidence of steatorrhoea at all. If malabsorption is suspected, barium studies of the stomach and small bowel are required, and these can be organized from general practice, as also can a faecal fat estimation if the patient is co-operative. If a jejunal biopsy is necessary, however, this is best undertaken in a hospital setting, even if only as a day case.

In many elderly people malabsorption is a consequence of a previous partial gastrectomy and associated blind-loop syndrome, but it may also be caused by one of the chronic diarrhoeas, such as Crohn's disease, or small-bowel diverticula.

It must not be forgotten, and should be considered before embarking upon additional investigations, that malabsorption can occur as a result of the medications a patient is taking. Drugs that are sometimes involved include broad-spectrum antibiotics, some purgatives, e.g. phenolphthalein, and para-aminosalicylic acid (PAS). There are also of course other conditions, such as long-standing congestive cardiac failure and coeliac disease, although the latter is rarely diagnosed for the first time in old age.

Treatment is centred around correcting the underlying abnormality and replacing the nutritional deficiencies. In many instances, it is impossible for this to be organized without further referral.

Malnutrition

The Department of Health and Social Security carried out a nutritional survey of old people at home, following a cohort of 483 people aged over 70, over a five-year period. As with other diseases, the prevalence of malnutrition rose with age, and 12 per cent of the men and 8 per cent of the women were malnourished.

The survey revealed two sets of results that are helpful to the person trying to assess the nutritional status of an old person in his own home. The first was that malnutrition was associated with certain medical and social conditions and that these could be regarded as risk factors for malnutrition. If one or more is present, malnutrition should be suspected and excluded.

The second set of findings which were helpful was the distinction between physical signs which were associated with malnutrition to a statistically significant degree from those which were not.

Table 7.3 Medical and social conditions associated with malnutrition

Condition	Special feature of malnutrition associated with condition, in addition to generalized malnutrition
Partial gastrectomy	Nutritional anaemia
Chronic bronchitis and emphysema	
Confusion	
Depression	
Edentulous and failure to use dentures	Fibre deficiency, constipation, and incontinence
Difficulty in swallowing	Vitamin D deficiency
Housebound	
No regular cooked meals	
In social class IV or V	
In receipt of supplementary benefits	

Physical signs significantly associated with malnutrition

   Wasted appearance
   Sublingual haemorrhage
   Sublingual varicosities
   Red seborrhoeic nasolabial folds
   Hyperkeratosis
   Inappropriate pigmentation of exposed skin

In this study a smooth atrophic tongue, flat nails and koilonychia, angular stomatitis, and cheilosis were not associated with malnutrition.

It is often difficult to confirm a history of dietary inadequacy from the people affected themselves, and it may be necessary to seek confirmation from a reliable third party. Examination will often indicate the consequences of nutritional deficiencies, such as the classical changes of iron deficiency and an anaemia, and the signs of vitamin B_{12} deficiency. There will also be biochemical evidence, and it is not uncommon to find a low serum albumin, signs of osteomalacia, i.e. a low calcium, and an elevated alkaline phosphatase. A routine blood count will also show evidence of anaemia which is usually hypochromic and microcytic. If these abnormalities are present, but the dietary intake appears to be adequate then it is necessary to consider the possibility of malabsorption as described in more detail above.

This problem is remedied by prescribing the appropriate vitamin supplements, considering the necessity for meals on wheels or attendance at a lunch club, and referring the problem to the social worker and relatives so that the underlying difficulties which have led to a deficient diet can be tackled. If the weight loss or biochemical abnormalities continue, it is probable that there is another factor involved and further investigation is necessary.

Dental problems   One of the reasons why some older people do not eat enough is that they have difficulty with eating meat, vegetables, and foods with a high content of cereal fibre, either because their teeth or gums are painful, or because their dentures are ill-fitting and cause them pain. Like younger people, old people should consult a dentist regularly whether or not they have symptoms, and they should also seek help promptly when they develop symptoms. Those with teeth should see their dentist at least once a year. Those who have dentures should consult a dentist every second year, provided that they do not develop symptoms in between these check-ups. Unfortunately many old people do not see a dentist as often as this for three reasons:

1 The low expectations of older people, their relatives, and professional people.
2 Their immobility (see p. 93).
3 The increasing difficulty in which people have finding a dentist willing to treat them 'on the NHS'.

If a personal approach to a friend who is a dentist is of no avail, it is worth while seeking the advice of the District Dental Officer,and it may be worth while asking whether an old person could be seen by the dentist who visits the day hospital, even if he has no medical need for day hospital attendance.

Myocardial infarction

The treatment of myocardial infarction and the importance of risk factors in the elderly is similar to that in younger patients. There are, however, one or two specific issues that are worth mentioning, and these are summarized below.

The need to admit to hospital

It is now generally accepted that many patients, especially the elderly, with a myocardial infarction do not require hospital treatment. Many elderly patients in particular do not wish to be sent to hospital, and in an uncomplicated myocardial infarction it is very reasonable to treat the patient at home. A patient who is shocked, however, who develops an arrhythmia, or who is found to be in heart failure should be admitted to hospital as soon as possible. It will also be necessary to admit any patient who lives on their own, or otherwise has nobody to care for them.

As the use of streptokinase and similar drugs is proving to be of benefit, this may change current practice, and some elderly patients may require hospital admission for such therapy.

Analgesia

Many of our elders develop myocardial infarction without pain, and if present it is often not very severe. Diamorphine or morphine with an antiemetic may be necessary, but it is often possible to prescribe a milder preparation. Whatever the circumstances prompt pain relief is extremely important.

Bed-rest

Mobilization of an elderly patient following a myocardial infarction is usually started the day after the infarction as long as there are no complications and the patient is pain-free. Initially this takes place slowly and gradually, increasing over a period of a week to ten days. The reappearance or persistence of pain, or the development of heart failure or an arrhythmia indicates the need to return the patient to bed, even though there is a risk of developing a DVT and the other consequences of bed-rest in the elderly.

If it is necessary to treat cardiac failure or arrhythmia at home, a standard therapeutic approach should be used. It must be remembered though that small doses of the drug should be tried initially, and that a loop-diuretic (i.e. frusemide or bumetanide) should only be used to promote an urgent diuresis. If the patient's recovery does not prove to be as straightforward as originally anticipated, referral to hospital is usually necessary.

Oedema of the ankles

Most people who present with simple ankle oedema are unlikely to require diuretics. One should not assume that it is a symptom of cardiac failure unless there is other clinical evidence to support this, e.g. an elevated JVP, bilateral basal crepitations, or a third heart sound. If it is in fact due to heart failure, as well as treating this it is important to look for any underlying cause for the onset of the cardiac failure, since occasionally a treatable condition will be discovered. Although ischaemic heart disease is by far the commonest cause, hypertension, valvular heart disease, and anaemia not infrequently cause cardiac failure in the elderly.

Other causes of ankle oedema include the following.

1 *Immobility*: Although this may be unilateral, e.g. after a cerebrovascular accident, when it may be aggravated by diminishing venous tone, or a

DVT, odema due to generalized immobility is more frequently bilateral and is due to a combination of the effects of gravity and the lack of muscle pump action.

2 *Hypoproteinaemia*: This essentially means a low serum albumin, for which there are many potential causes. These include liver disease, inadequate nutrition, malabsorption, and less commonly the nephrotic syndrome.

3 *Drugs*: Among those pharmaceutical preparations which cause fluid retention, the most commonly used include steroids (especially corticosteroids and stilboestrol), carbenoxolone sodium, and non-steroidal anti-inflammatory drugs.

4 *Venous obstruction*: Thrombosis in the deep veins of the legs occur far more commonly than is suspected and should be carefully watched for after a cerebrovascular accident or a coronary thrombosis, and in people with neoplastic disease. Deep venous thromboses are also a post-operative hazard in people who have recently undergone surgery, and with the trend towards ever earlier discharge home post-operatively for many procedures, this has to be borne in mind. Typically unilateral, they can of course occur bilaterally, although bilateral ankle oedema is more commonly secondary to venous obstruction in the pelvic veins or inferior vena cava. The latter may be precipitated not only by an abdominal mass, but also by ascites.

Beware of confusing a DVT with a ruptured Baker's cyst. The latter is quite common (and may co-exist with a DVT).

Varicose veins are also associated with ankle oedema in some patients, and in these cases it is the increase in pressure in the column of blood in the vessels rather than thrombosis that is responsible.

5 *Lymphatic obstruction*: This most commonly arises as a result of neoplastic deposits in lymph nodes. It is then often unilateral.

Occasionally, one comes across a patient with Milroy's disease in which there is a congenital absence of lymphatics; but they will have had swollen legs for most of their life and are unlikely to present with it as a problem for the first time in old age.

It is also important not to forget that the constrictive effects of some clothes can result in venous stasis and an aggravation of ankle oedema. An example of this is the elasticated legging of old ladies' underwear, and the practice often employed of keeping stockings in position by twisting their tops. These are not always obvious after the patient has been undressed by a nurse ready for examination. They are rarely, however, responsible for more than a little fluid accumulation.

Investigation   The causes of ankle oedema is usually apparent from a careful history and examination supported by a full blood count, and estimation of urea and electrolytes together with a biochemical screen. If a more serious condition is suspected, or a DVT, referral to hospital is necessary, but in many cases treatment can be instituted without further investigation.

Management

1 The first step of course is to treat any underlying condition if this is possible.
2 The next practical step is to elevate the foot of the bed at night in order to re-distribute the oedema. This is not appropriate, however, if the patient is suffering with (a) cardiac failure because of the risk of orthopnea, (b) oesophageal reflux secondary to a hiatus hernia, or (c) in someone with peripheral arterial disease. Simple advice to raise the legs often leads to them being put on a pouffe, resting on the calves. This is bad for the venous return—and does not help as the leg is still dependent. It is better to advise the patient to sit sideways on a settee, with his or her heel on its padded arm.
3 *Supportive treatment.* Crêpe bandages are unsatisfactory in the elderly in many cases because they can be very difficult for an old person to put on properly. Elastic stockings are often advocated, but they too can be a struggle to wear, and in some cases tubigrip-type stockinet will suffice as a second-best option. Exercising ankles and knees may help.

Useful advice for elderly patients and their relatives

The correct use of elastic stockings (graduated support hosiery)

Put the stockings on in bed, *before* you get up in the morning. If you have difficulty putting the stockings on, try:

- Wearing rubber gloves to increase grip
- Sprinkling the legs with talc
- Putting a pair of tights on first: This makes it easier to roll on the elastic stockings, by lowering friction

Hand-wash the stockings in warm, not hot, water. Do not hang them out to dry in direct sunlight: they will lose their elasticity.

Osteomalacia

Osteomalacia differs from osteoporosis because of a deficiency of calcification of the normal bone matrix of osteoid. It is most commonly caused by vitamin D deficiency of a dietary origin, or in consequence of malabsorption. In some cases, especially in immigrant populations, it has been described in relation to lack of exposure to sunlight, and may also be a feature of renal disease, since vitamin D metabolism is impaired in the presence of chronic renal failure. Certain drugs, especially anticonvulsants, also interfere with vitamin D metabolism in the liver and can precipitate osteomalacia.

Presentation

The presenting features may be non-specific in nature and consist of vague reports of weakness and aches and pains. These should be taken seriously, especially if they are accompanied by difficulty in performing normal daily activities such as climbing stairs. Osteomalacia is characterized by proximal muscle weakness as well as the skeletal deformities resulting from softening of the bones themselves, resulting in features such as the kyphosis so often seen.

Investigations

An X-ray is helpful in confirming the diagnosis, since not only will it reveal generalized decalcification, but possibly also the pseudofractures known as Looser's zones, which are areas of decalcification presenting as apparent cracks in the cortex and best seen in the axillary border of the scapula, the femoral neck, and the upper end of the humerus amongst other sites. This finding is diagnostic.

Biochemical abnormalities include a raised alkaline phosphatase, a calcium that is often low, but may be normal, and a low phosphate. The calcium and phosphate levels respond rapidly to treatment even if this consists only of a hospital diet with an adequate vitamin D intake. Diagnosis can therefore be difficult on occasion unless Looser's zones are found on the X-ray, or a bone biopsy is performed.

Treatment

This is oral or intramuscular vitamin D in the standard doses, i.e. 1500–5000 iu daily for 2–3 months, and following resolution of the condition, prophylactic treatment with 500 iu daily (which is contained in one Calcium-with-Vitamin D Tablet). Calcium supplements are also required in many cases, especially initially. All patients on vitamin D and/or calcium should have their renal function and plasma calcium levels monitored regularly (weekly, initially).

An underlying cause should be sought and where appropriate treated. If this can be remedied long-term vitamin and calcium supplements may be avoided, although initially necessary. The calcium and phosphate levels may return to normal rapidly, but the alkaline phosphatase will take much longer to return to normal.

Osteoporosis

Osteoporosis is caused by a loss of bone substance, i.e. both protein, matrix, and calcium salts, the substance left being fully mineralized unless there is concurrent osteomalacia, which not infrequently occurs in older patients. Its presence should be suspected when the typical symptoms present in any patient with a predisposing medical history including Cushing's disease and steroid therapy, rheumatoid arthritis, and immobilization. Perhaps the commonest presenting symptom is back pain associated with a collapsed vertebral body, or fracture of a bone elsewhere, as in the femoral neck or a Colles' fracture of the wrist.

For practical purposes the diagnosis can be made radiologically, but where there is doubt, e.g. where it may have important consequences on the further management of a patient on steroids, or the possibility of concurrent osteomalacia exists, hospital referral for bone biopsy is usually necessary. In pure osteoporosis there are no abnormalities in the plasma calcium, phosphate, and alkaline phosphatase.

Treatment is controversial and probably ineffective, and as usual preventive measures are best, although this is not always possible. Anabolic steroids, calcium supplements, and vitamin D analogues have all been advocated, but the best treatment is still a matter of debate, at least in old age. There is, however, good evidence that hormone replacement therapy, or calcium supplementation, started in the early post menopausal years may have preventive value. It is certainly worth advising the patient to use her skeleton as much as possible—e.g. walking; gardening; cycling; 'keep fit' exercises.

Paget's disease of bone

The majority of cases of Paget's disease need no treatment or further consideration. It usually affects one or occasionally two or three bones in a particular patient, and most patients remain symptomless. Occasionally phenomena such as deafness, headaches, and bone pain arise, and even the need to purchase a larger size hat if the disease is localized to the skull. Complications include pathological fractures and rarely, but significantly, sarcomatous change. High-output cardiac failure and compression of the spinal cord can occur, but are only seen infrequently. The finding of Paget's disease as an incidental abnormality on an X-ray in a symptomless patient is probably best ignored, but the diagnosis noted in case relevant symptoms emerge at a later date.

Investigation

It is characterized by normal calcium and phosphate levels unless the patient is immobile, when the calcium may rise. The alkaline phosphatase is usually elevated, often to quite high levels when the disease is active; and it is not infrequently diagnosed in this way, i.e. investigation of an incidental finding of a high alkaline phosphatase on a biochemical screen.

Treatment

Initially this is symptomatic, and simple analgesics are probably best for pain and discomfort. Calcitonin is also used for pain that does not respond to simple analgesics and when some of the neurological complications ensue, but it has to be given intramuscularly for several months and is probably best initially supervised via a hospital outpatient clinic. Diphosphonates are also helpful in some cases.

Parkinsonism

The classical features of parkinsonism are too well known to merit detailed consideration here, but it is important to emphasize the effects of the bradykinesia. This can lead to great difficulty in rising from a chair or getting out of bed, which is often misinterpreted as laziness or awkwardness by others when they see the patient walking on another occasion. This point needs explaining to relatives so that the patient is not unnecessarily maligned.

The first and probably most important step when considering parkinsonism in the elderly is to eliminate the side-effects of phenothiazine or related drugs as its cause. It is extremely common, both in hospital and outside, to discover patients taking a drug which induces extrapyramidal side-effects and an antiparkinsonian agent concurrently to counteract these effects, without the relationship between the two being appreciated by the doctor responsible. In the majority of instances the drugs involved can easily be discontinued or reduced in dosage to obviate the need for antiparkinsonian therapy, which in its turn introduces additional and often very disabling side-effects of its own. In addition, in many such instances the symptoms are being treated with an L-dopa preparation, which is clearly inappropriate when the rigidity and other signs are phenothiazine-induced, since these drugs produce parkinsonism by blocking the receptor sites for dopamine within the basal ganglia. Prescribing an L-dopa combination preparation in an attempt to increase the concentration of dopamine at the appropriate sites does not often significantly improve matters. If it is impossible to withdraw the offending drug completely or reduce its dosage sufficiently to make antiparkinsonian treatment unnecessary, one of the anticholinergic preparations should be prescribed, e.g. benzhexol or orphenadrine.

The L-dopa combination preparations, usually L-dopa and carbidopa or L-dopa and benserazide, are probably the most effective drugs in the elderly for the treatment of Parkinson's disease. They are more effective in controlling the bradykinesia and rigidity than in relieving the tremor. Since dopamine is an active transmitter at other sites within and outside the brain, side-effects are common, particularly with larger doses. For this reason it is important to start with the smallest possible dose and slowly work up, taking care to watch out for the onset of gastrointestinal upset, depression, hallucinations, and confusional states. It is also necessary in people on L-dopa preparations to watch out for the 'on–off effect' which occurs in a small number of patients after long-term treatment. This is marked by rapid intermittent dyskinesia. It may be helped by prescribing small doses of levo-dopa more frequently, the precise timing of each dose being determined by trial and error. The monoamine oxidase B inhibitor selegilene (5–10 mg/24 h PO) may be very helpful, and does not cause episodes of hypertension. Also consider bromocriptine (e.g. 2.5 mg *nocte*) to reduce morning dystonias.

Evidence is accumulating that selegiline 10 mg/24 hours by mouth delays disease progression, making it appear to be an attractive agent to consider *before* the use of L-dopa. Selegiline (Eldepryl) is a type B-selective monoamine oxidase inhibitor and has virtually no adverse pressor effects. Basic clinical studies suggest that the activity of monoamine oxidase and the formation of free radicals predispose patients to nigral degeneration and contribute to the emergence and progression of Parkinson's disease. The Parkinsonian Study Group (1989) in Rochester, New York, has found that selegiline appears to delay the progression of Parkinson's disease and the need for L-dopa, and significantly reduces the risk of having to give up full-time employment. Twenty-four per cent of patients receiving selegiline deteriorated over one year so that L-dopa had to be started, compared with 44 per cent who did not receive selegiline.

The other major group of drugs used in the treatment of parkinsonism are the anticholinergic compounds, which have been in use for over a century. Among this group are benzhexol, which is extremely effective but produces confusion in a large number of elderly patients, and orphenadrine. Other side-effects include postural hypotension, and the aggravation of any tendency towards glaucoma or towards retention of urine in men with prostatic hypertrophy.

Amantadine is rarely used in the treatment of Parkinson's disease, or parkinsonism in the elderly, but it is worth considering when the other preparations have to be discontinued. It is generally better tolerated, but unfortunately it is not so effective. Amongst its side-effects are confusion and fluid retention.

In some patients a combination of drugs is helpful, for example the patient whose salivation may be controlled with a small dose of an anticholinergic agent while an L-dopa preparation is used as a major therapeutic agent. It is also worth adding small doses of anticholinergic drugs to the treatment in a patient in whom L-dopa preparations have not produced a satisfactory result.

Pressure sores

Most people are familiar with the risk to an immobile patient of developing pressure sores in the sacral area, over the greater trochanter, and over the heels. It is often forgotten, however, that underlying conditions may aggravate a tendency to pressure sores and should be sought in any patient in whom there is a likelihood of these developing. Their presence not only alerts one to the increased risk of a particular patient developing an area of breakdown, but, since some of them are amenable to treatment, identification may be helpful in reducing the risk of a sore occurring, or possibly limiting its severity. These factors include hypotension and peripheral vascular disease, as well as malnutrition, anaemia, and urinary or faecal incontinence. Apart from these additional risk factors, pressure sores are particularly likely to arise in any patient who is immobile for any length of time.

Treatment

Any predisposing factor or underlying condition should obviously be treated if this is possible. Catheterization may also help if it is considered that urinary incontinence is aggravating the situation. The mainstay of treatment, however, is regular turning, preferably every two hours; and for this reason a patient in whom pressure sores have arisen may well have to be admitted to hospital. Sheepskin heel pads, ripple mattresses, and other similar aids are useful agents in prevention but where healing is concerned come second-best to regular turning and keeping the patient off his pressure area.

Semipermiable adhesive film dressings (e.g. *Tegaderm*®) may be helpful in areas where there are incipient pressure sores.

The role of infection is often misunderstood, and since it is usually superficial, it is probably best treated with local antiseptic measures rather than systemic or local antibiotics. If there is severe local cellulitis involving deeper tissues, systemic antibiotics are probably necessary; but a swab should be taken first to indicate which is the most appropriate antibiotic.

If there is dead or necrotic tissue in the centre of the sore, this must be removed either surgically or using an enzyme preparation before there is any chance of the wound healing. Again this is probably easier in hospital, but could easily be undertaken in a community or cottage hospital rather than a district general hospital or geriatric unit. If a sore takes a long time to heal an opinion from a plastic surgeon is worth while; and it is important to remember if the breakdown has occurred over a bony prominence that there may be infection in the underlying bone. This will usually become apparent radiologically.

Many different agents have been advocated to enhance healing, including maggots, insulin and egg white, oxygen, and sugar, but these probably play only a secondary part if any, regular turning and keeping the patient off the pressure area being the mainstay of treatment. Ultraviolet light is possibly one exception to this and is occasionally helpful in promoting granulation tissue and possibly retarding bacterial overgrowth.

Other measures, especially attention to the patient's state of nutrition, topical preparations containing streptokinase and similar enzymes, and other preparations marketed for local application are occasionally helpful. They are too numerous to mention in detail. A similar approach to local toilet as mentioned in the discussion of leg ulcers is also essential (p. 109).

Renal impairment

Elevation of blood urea

Many elderly people have a blood urea level that is within the normal limits for younger people, i.e. less than 7 mmol/l. Not infrequently, however, it is found to be as high as 10 mmol/l without any evidence of a significant underlying pathology. It is not unreasonable to accept this as normal, but a level greater than 10 always requires further consideration. It is probably best to exclude dehydration, which will usually be clinically obvious, in the first instance. Dryness of the mouth, tachycardia, reduced skin turgor, and diminished urinary output all indicate dehydration, especially if there is an elevated specific gravity in the urine. The serum creatinine level may also be proportionately lower than the urea, but in the elderly the creatinine can rise as a direct result of dehydration, although this is generally not appreciated. The presence of dehydration can also be surmised by finding an elevated haematocrit and raised serum protein level. The commonest causes include diuretic treatment and pyrexial illness, although any elderly person taking to their bed may reduce their fluid intake.

An increase in protein breakdown, as may occur for instance after an upper gastrointestinal haemorrhage, can also elevate the blood urea; but this is usually a short-term phenomenon. There is in any case usually supportive evidence indicating that bleeding has occurred. More commonly, however, increased protein breakdown is a non-specific phenomenon occurring in many illnesses and can also be associated with the use of some drugs, for instance steroids and tetracycline derivatives, as well as being an accompaniment of many fevers. If either of these two conditions, i.e. dehydration or increased protein breakdown, is considered to be the cause of the elevated urea then a repeat estimation when the underlying condition has been corrected should confirm that further investigation is unnecessary.

Chronic renal failure

In chronic renal failure there will be an elevated serum phosphate and uric acid and a low serum calcium. The patient will usually be acidotic with a low serum bicarbonate, and the potassium may rise. A normochromic anaemia is usually present, often falling to as low as 7 or 8 g per cent. It is surprising how quickly a low haemoglobin can be produced in renal disease, however, and such a low level does not necessarily imply that the duration of the renal failure should be measured in months, since it could well be weeks. Detecting protein in the urine will also indicate the presence of kidney damage. If chronic renal failure is suspected it is extremely important to look for any treatable underlying aetiological factors, including a high blood pressure and diabetes mellitus. Controlling both these conditions may well delay further deterioration in renal function. There are other conditions that need excluding, and these include prostatic hypertrophy, or obstruction due to stones or more rarely urethral valves. There are of course many chronic conditions for which there is little available treatment, and these include chronic pyelonephritis, nephrosclerosis, and diabetic nephropathy.

In addition to the investigations mentioned above it is important to arrange the examination of a fresh specimen of urine and an abdominal ultrasound scan. Occasionally, a sterile pyuria is discovered, and although this in theory indicates the possibility of renal tract tuberculosis it is not uncommonly due to a partially treated lower urinary tract infection. Intravenous urography (IVU) may also be necessary even if a high-dose infusion method has to be employed. A patient with chronic renal failure referred to a hospital clinic for further investigation will usually be screened for myeloma and collagenoses, as treatment of these conditions is usually worth while. There is, however, no reason why all these investigations should not be carried out from the general practice setting.

Amyloid is an uncommon cause of chronic renal failure in the elderly, but is more likely to occur in an older person than in the younger patient. It should be suspected if the renal failure is accompanied by normal-size or slightly enlarged kidneys.

Treatment of chronic renal failure is probably best carried out in the hospital environment, although this does not necessarily need district general hospital facilities. There is little difference between the treatment in younger and older patients, the principles being the same, i.e. controlling fluid and electrolyte balance, correcting the acidosis, and restricting protein intake. It is necessary to avoid infection and dehydration if at all possible, but a high index of suspicion should be maintained for both of these conditions, since early detection and treatment will often avoid or limit a further reduction in renal function.

Acute renal failure

Acute renal failure in older people is usually of the acute-on-chronic type. This is indicated by finding the characteristic biochemical and haemato-logical abnormalities already described. Admission to hospital is necessary if it is decided that the condition ought to be treated rather than be allowed to run its natural course in a patient where this is appropriate. The principles of treatment include controlling fluid and electrolyte balance, a high-calorie low-protein diet, vitamin supplements, and sometimes anabolic steroids. If a decision is made to try to treat the patient outside the context of a district general hospital, in addition to the points already mentioned it is particularly important to avoid over-hydration, which can result in cardiac failure. Although a severe anaemia should be corrected it must be remembered that there is a high potassium and protein content in stored blood. A patient with moderate anaemia is probably best left untransfused. The other pitfalls to avoid are those of infection, dehydration, and urinary tract obstruction, just as in the case of chronic renal failure.

Diagnosis of the underlying pathology is probably most efficiently made in hospital. Since some of the causes of acute renal failure are eminently treatable it is important that this is taken into account when a decision is made about the patient's management.

Associated abnormalities in the urine

Proteinuria Occasionally proteinuria is caused by contamination, for instance by vaginal secretions in women. Unless there is other frank evidence of renal tract disease, it is important to exclude contamination as a cause of proteineuria before investigating the condition further. Microscopy may reveal vaginal cells, confirming contamination from this source. It may also be excluded by carefully repeating the test, taking as great care as possible to avoid contamination, although this can be difficult in elderly women.

The commonest cause of proteinuria is probably a lower urinary tract infection. The accompanying bacterial growth and the presence of leucocytes will make the diagnosis obvious, even if typical symptoms are not present. It is also important to consider the possibility of an underlying cause, since urinary tract infections, particularly if recurrent, may be caused or exacerbated by underlying pathology.

Having excluded contamination or a lower urinary tract infection, the next step is to consider those conditions associated with chronic renal failure. If chronic renal failure is present there may be other evidence of renal damage in the urine, for instance casts and red and white blood cells, in addition to the biochemical markers of impaired renal function described above.

Although it occurs uncommonly in older people, the nephrotic syndrome is also a cause of proteinuria. It may occur more frequently than is generally appreciated. It is sometimes caused by minimal change lesions which will respond to treatment with prednisolone, but it is more usually a concomitant of systemic diseases such as diabetes mellitus, collagenoses, malignancy, and more rarely renal vein thrombosis. A degree of nephrotic syndrome may accompany chronic congestive cardiac failure. This condition, i.e. nephrotic syndrome, should be excluded in a patient presenting with heavy proteinuria, peripheral oedema, and hypoproteinaemia. The serum cholesterol may also be elevated. Hospital referral is indicated if it is suspected.

Asymptomatic bacteriuria This is not an infrequent finding in elderly people and can pose problems in deciding whether or not treatment is appropriate. It is commonly associated with chronic pyelonephritis, and most authorities would probably agree that treatment is harmful and unnecessary unless symptoms develop or renal function is deteriorating. This is also true of the catheterized patient.

Sexual dysfunction and sexually transmitted diseases

Sexual activity is an important facet in the lives of many elderly people (Kellett 1989). It is important to be aware of problems such as impotence, which are common side-effects of drugs such as antihypertensives. Some authorities insist that patients be told of these side-effects before treatment is started. Others realize that a more subtle approach may be justifiable— because warnings of impotence and other anxiety-related dysfunctions may become self-fulfilling prophecies. In one study of elderly patients (>70 years old) undergoing gynaecological surgery, more than a third were sexually active (Lawton and Hacker 1989). This underlines the importance of pre-operative counselling.

In another study (Rogstad and Bignell 1989) more than a quarter of elderly patients (>60 years old) attending a genitourinary department had multiple regular sexual partners (up to 30 in the last six months). About the same proportion of patients had sexually transmitted diseases—thereby showing how wrong it is to discount the possibility of sexually transmitted diseases on the grounds of age.

Subdural haematoma

This is a condition which is commonly diagnosed at post-mortem, since although the symptoms may be apparent shortly following an obvious inj y. it is extremely common for the trauma responsible to be minor or forgot and in the past. Classically it presents as fluctuating signs and sympton especially a fluctuating level of consciousness. Other presentations include a fluctuating hemiplegia or other neurological signs, as well as m. non-specific symptoms such as headache. As in the cases of tuberculor subacute bacterial endocarditis, and hypothyroidism, it is a condition which a high index of suspicion must always be maintained when dealing v elderly patients, and since treatment may result in considerable improv ment, further investigation is always necessary. This is best arranged in the context of a short hospital admission, which is often necessary in any case on account of the presenting disabilities. Where a patient is confined to a community hospital with radiological expertise a skull X-ray may reveal shift of mid-line structures and make the diagnosis more likely. If this is found, referral to the local neurosurgical centre is necessary for further confirmation and consideration of evacuation of the underlying haematoma. In any case in which there is doubt, hospital referral is necessary.

Thyroid disorders

Hypothyroidism

Although all doctors know that hypothyroidism is often non-specific in its presentation in older patients and is therefore easily missed, the diagnosis is still not made in many cases and may elude even the keenest practitioner or geriatrician. In the elderly it most commonly follows previous thyroid ablation or occurs as an idiopathic condition. The iatrogenic type may either be after surgery, when it is said that nearly 50 per cent of patients become hypothyroid within a year of partial thyroidectomy, or after radioactive iodine therapy, when 80 per cent of patients are said to become hypothyroid within 15 years. The incidence is therefore very high following either procedure on the thyroid gland and should really be watched for rather than merely being picked up somewhat opportunistically.

Other causes include overdosage with antithyroid drugs, as well as from other non-related compounds, e.g. lithium carbonate and amiodarone. Hypopituitarism is rare in the elderly, as is autoimmune thyroiditis too. Nevertheless these conditions should be considered if it is not possible to explain the thyroid malfunction on other grounds. Autoimmune thyroiditis should particularly be considered if there is already a pre-existing autoimmune disorder such as pernicious anaemia, Addison's disease (of the idiopathic type), or vitiligo, whilst hypopituitarism is usually associated with evidence of loss of other trophic hormones. In both the latter, hospital referral is necessary for confirmation of the diagnosis.

Clinical features These are the same at any age and do not merit detailed consideration here. There are, however, one or two points that are worth emphasizing. In the first place some of the classic features of hypothyroidism are a normal finding in many of the elderly, e.g. loss of the outer third of the eyebrows and constipation, but they should nevertheless alert one to look for other signs. Particularly useful are the bradycardia in a patient who is not being treated concurrently with beta-blockers or some other drugs which could produce this, and the slowly relaxing reflexes. It must be stressed that it is the relaxation phase that is important, and although it is usual to seek this sign with the ankle jerk, the biceps reflex is often better in older people.

Investigations Diagnosis can only be confirmed biochemically and the most useful investigation is the serum TSH level, which is usually greater than 6 mu/l in primary hypothyroidism. The T3 level is unhelpful, since a failing thyroid gland will often secrete more T3 than normal. Occasionally, however, one is still uncertain, and at this point it is probably best to refer the patient to hospital for a TRH test (thyrotrophin releasing hormone test), although this could be undertaken from general practice.

Thyroid hormone levels may be altered by other factors, such as oestrogen therapy and phenothiazine administration if this is prolonged, and in hypoproteinaemic states, since 99 per cent of the hormones are protein-bound. If the TSH level is elevated, but the T4 level is within the normal range, it is not always necessary to conclude that the patient has hypothyroid-ism since the TSH may be elevated in an attempt to 'drive' a failing thyroid gland. Under these circumstances the patient should be carefully followed up, since there is a higher risk of hypothyroidism, and this is particularly so if there has been previous treatment of thyrotoxicosis.

Treatment When treating the elderly it is essential to start with the lowest possible dose of thyroxine, and never more than 0.05 mg a day, or even half this dose if heart failure is present. They are very sensitive to exogenous thyroxine and there is always a risk of precipitating myocardial infarction. Thyroxine takes three to four days to begin work, with maximum response after a further week or so. Assuming that the initial dose is tolerated, it can be doubled at two-week intervals until a maximum of 0.2 mg a day is being taken. Very occasionally 0.3 mg will be necessary, but the correct dose is that which returns the T4 and TSH to normal values. It can then be monitored on clinical symptoms and signs, e.g. weight loss, tachycardia, heat intolerance, etc. and the T3 (triiodothyronine) level estimated if there is any evidence of early thyrotoxicosis. Since this is often a test which takes a week or two before the answer is available, it is probably best to ease back a little on the thyroxine dosage if there is objective clinical evidence of thyrotoxicosis.

Thyrotoxicosis

As is the case with myxoedema, thyrotoxicosis does not always present in the elderly with classical symptoms and signs. Indeed it is possible for the initial presentation to be one of apathy. Both the serum triiodothyronine (T3) and thyroxine (T4) are raised in most patients who are thyrotoxic, although some patients may have T3 thyrotoxicosis only and an even smaller number an elevation of thyroxine alone. An estimate of the plasma TSH level by radioimmunoassay technique is probably the best means of diagnosing the majority of thyrotoxic patients. It is also helpful in indicating which patients are relapsing into thyrotoxicosis after being treated.

The thyrotrophin-releasing hormone (TRH) test is occasionally necessary when investigating thyroid disease. Although this is usually performed in a hospital outpatient department, there is no reason why it could not be done in the general practitioner's surgery in the few cases where it is necessary. After blood has been taken to allow the basal TSH level to be measured, 200 micrograms of TRH are injected intravenously and blood samples taken for subsequent estimates of TSH level 20 minutes after the injection. There is normally a peak response at about 20 minutes, but this is suppressed in thyrotoxicosis since the raised level of thyroid hormones in the blood inhibit the release of TSH. This response, however, may also be affected by certain drugs, including L-dopa, corticosteroids, and also thyroxine if the dose is above 0.2 mg daily. Abnormal pituitary function will also prevent a response to the injection.

Treatment It is probably best to treat elderly people with thyrotoxicosis with radioactive iodine and subsequent thyroid-hormone replacement. Antithyroid drugs (carbimazole or propylthiouracil) may give useful control, but need to be stopped well before the dose of radioactive iodine is given.

In addition, many of the features of thyrotoxicosis will respond to treatment with beta-blockers, although they will have little effect on diarrhoea, weight loss, or eye signs. These can be discontinued when the thyrotoxicosis has been brought under control. Thyroid function tests should be monitored routinely, e.g. every three to six months, until the patient is satisfactorily treated with replacement therapy.

Tuberculosis

The dramatic drop in the incidence of tuberculosis in younger people has not been mirrored to the same extent in the elderly, mainly because so many of them have quiescent tuberculosis acquired in their youth. Reactivation of this primary infection is the commonest problem.

Presentation   This is often non-specific, with ill-defined illness and general deterioration in health. It is easy to assume that it is secondary to an incurable wasting illness such as a neoplasm, which then makes further investigation of the patient less likely. It should therefore be considered a possibility in any patient with unexplained malaise, anorexia, weight loss, and fever, as well as the more classical presentations such as persistent or recurrent chest infections and ascites. In our own practice over the last five years the most common non-pulmonary presentation has been after the use of steroids (usually injected by rheumatologists into joints) or as sterile pyuria. The main lesson to learn is that once a patient has had TB, never think that he or she is 100 per cent cured—and avoid ster~· ' unless essential, and if they are used (after explaining the risks to the patient), the patient should be monitored closely, with TB uppermost in everyone's mind.

A chest X-ray may help confirm the diagnosis, but all too often all one finds is the pre-existing changes indicating infection many years ago. Unless there is existing cavitation or miliary mottling, the chest X-ray may not be helpful. If a patient in whom tuberculosis is suspected is producing sputum, a sample should be sent for microscopy and culture, and the possibility of tuberculosis should be specifically mentioned on the request card. It can also be helpful to re-X-ray a chest of doubtful significance six to eight weeks later in order to see if there has been any change, if there are no previous X-rays with which to compare the present film. A sterile pyuria indicates the possibility of renal tract TB, and early morning urine specimens should be examined, as well as arranging an IVU and abdominal ultrasound scan.

Where the index of suspicion is high the patient should be referred to hospital for further investigation, and this should always be the case if there is a pleural effusion or ascites, since these can be tapped and and an appropriate specimen can be sent for microscopy and culture.

Tuberculin test   This is of doubtful value in the elderly, since its interpretation is very difficult. Often a positive reaction only reflects previous infection rather than indicating present activity. The latter may be suspected if the reaction is extremely positive, however; but in so many cases it is not so. If the reaction is negative, active infection is unlikely unless the patient is the subject of an overwhelming infection, which will be apparent on clinical grounds. A negative reaction in the presence of active disease also occurs in those who are immunosuppressed, e.g. by drugs or a lymphoma. Occasionally, however, the reaction remains negative even in the presence of active infection. It is therefore preferable to diagnose active tuberculosis more objectively; but a positive result from a low dose of tuberculin, e.g. 5 units in 0.1 ml of solution can be considered supportive evidence until proved otherwise if the size of the reaction is 10 mm or greater.

Treatment   This is similar to that in younger patients with one of the combination regimes, and these drugs are best initially prescribed under supervision in hospital. The three major worries in treating the elderly with tuberculosis are drug compliance, which is often low, retrobulbar neuritis as a side-effect of ethambutol, and a need to avoid giving streptomycin because of its high toxicity. In disseminated tuberculosis the GP has an important role in orchestrating the efforts of chest physicians, urologists, and microbiologists so as to ensure that the patient receives optimum treatment— without spending his or her entire life in the outpatient department.

Vertigo/giddiness/dizziness

These three symptoms are listed together since elderly people often have great difficulty in differentiating between them. They are also occasionally confused with the feeling of faintness, collapsing, and other synonyms. Before it is possible to elucidate any underlying cause, the doctor needs to know exactly what the patient is complaining of. Although it is by no means a counsel of perfection, it is easiest from a practical point of view to divide this problem into two different subgroups. In the first of these the patient experiences true vertigo with a rotational sensation, usually of the room or furniture going round him. In the other group this does not happen and the overwhelming sensation is one of instability, faintness, etc., but without any rotational component.

True vertigo

This can be produced simply by an accumulation of wax in the external auditory meatus, which is responsible more frequently than most appreciate. Middle-ear disease is also occasionally the cause in an older person, but disease of the auditory nerve, inner ear, cerebellum, and brainstem are probably commoner underlying factors. Brainstem-territory cerebrovascular disease is probably the commonest cause, with labyrinthitis and Ménière's disease following next. In the last-named there is a paroxysmal labrinthine disorder manifested as vertigo, deafness, and vomiting accompanied by tinnitus. Many other pathologies in this area, however, may be responsible, and this includes drug side-effects, e.g. over-dosage with aspirin. Since occasionally more sinister but remediable conditions such as an acoustic neuroma can present in this way, it is important to obtain a further opinion if a diagnosis cannot be made easily or the symptoms do not respond to the appropriate treatment.

Non-vertiginous giddiness/dizziness, etc.

As described above, this implies the absence of any rotational sensation. Vasovagal syncopal attacks occur in older people, occasionally for no reason, but before assuming this to be the case, it is important to exclude hypotension, whether postural or not, and anaemia. These pathologies always need further investigation. As in the case of true vertigo, disease of the brainstem, cerebellum, auditory nerve, and inner ear may also be involved.

Management   In many cases no underlying cause is discovered, whichever type of 'giddiness' it is, and in some it improves spontaneously. Although some with vertigo may have had a self-limiting condition such as a short attack of labyrinthitis, one is forced to accept the fact that little is presently understood about one of the more common disabling symptoms of the elderly. If the symptoms persist in a patient in whom there is no obvious underlying cause, he or she must be counselled on the need to take care when making a turn or other rotational movement, and when rising from the sitting or lying position. Many drugs are claimed to be of benefit and different regimes have different advocates. Experience shows, however, that different preparations seem to suit different patients for no objective reason, and although it is worth trying drugs such as antihistamines, mild phenothiazines, and betahistine, they should be discontinued if there is no objective evidence of improvement. This is particularly important because their side-effects may include phenomena which may aggravate a patient's original symptom, e.g. adding postural hypotension to their original presenting complaint. Referral to a geriatric or ENT clinic is necessary if an underlying condition is discovered which warrants this, or if troublesome symptoms persist.

Tinnitus is a common symptom which is often associated with vertigo, and can be extremely distressing. More than one in ten elderly people suffer with this problem at some stage. Referral for a further opinion is usually necessary, but often the only treatment possible is reassurance. This will help some sufferers, however, who associate it with an impending disaster, such as a stroke or inevitable deafness: but unfortunately many have to learn to tolerate it. Serious consideration should always be given to the underlying cause, since it may be the first sign of potentially treatable (or, at least, somewhat ameliorable) pathology, e.g. Ménière's disease and otosclerosis.

Visual impairment

There are so many potential causes of visual impairment in older people that it is not intended to try and cover them all, but rather to mention briefly those points which should be considered, especially in more elderly patients. There are two approaches to the consideration of loss of sight, either using a structure by structure appraisal starting at the front of the eyeball and working backwards, or the more practical clinical approach which will be used here. This divides the visual impairment into two major types, acute and chronic.

Acute loss of vision

Acute loss of vision is obviously an ophthalmological emergency. Severe pain in the eyes associated with vomiting in many instances and blurred vision from corneal oedema probably heralds an acute attack of angle-closure glaucoma. This should be further suspected if an oval dilated pupil fails to respond to light. In many patients there will have been previous subacute but self-limiting attacks.

   Immediate referral to an eye hospital casualty department is necessary for intensive pilocarpine and acetazolamide therapy or other medical treatment, and in the majority of cases probably drainage surgery.

   There are especially two retinal conditions which are associated with the sudden loss of vision. One of these is the detached retina and the other occlusive vascular disease affecting either the arterial or the venous system. Both should be referred to an Eye Department without delay (i.e. to be seen by an opthalmologist on the day they present). The history, e.g. features of giant cell arteritis or glaucoma, and examination of the eye, e.g. the retinal pallor and

---

Useful advice for elderly patients and their relatives on sight

Warning signs that need medical attention the same day

1 Persistent pain.
2 Sensitivity to light.
3 Seeing halos and rainbows around lights.
4 Flashing lights.
5 Loss of vision.
6 Double vision.
7 Redness and irritation.

'cherry red spot' of central or branch retinal arterial occlusion will often indicate that such an occlusion has occurred. However, the finer points of diagnosis and consideration of any underlying predisposing pathological entities are best left to the hospital.

Sometimes a patient claims to have lost vision in one or other eye when the lesion is really within the brain. The most frequent reason for this is probably the sudden onset of a homonymous hemianopia, which is interpreted by the patient as being caused by loss of sight in one or other eye. This may occur as a consequence of a cerebrovascular accident—when full examination will often reveal other localizing neurological signs, even if only of a mild nature. If any doubt exists however, a second opinion is necessary.

Chronic loss of vision

Slow onset of visual impairment is met with more frequently in older people than the acute and more urgent problems described above.

Cataract Cataract formation is common, and although in many people no underlying factors can be discovered, it is important to consider these, e.g. diabetes mellitus and long-term steroid therapy. If the cataract is unilateral and the other eye has normal or adequate vision, it is not necessary to consider cataract extraction unless there are other relevant factors, such as the onset of secondary glaucoma and other less common conditions. Cataract removal should be considered when vision is impaired to the extent that the activities of daily living are significantly affected, although the introduction of many modern techniques has resulted in a trend towards earlier surgical treatment.

Retinopathy Retinopathy, especially that of diabetes, is often discovered as an incidental finding when examining the fundus. In many patients, however, it contributes to visual impairment, as does the retinopathy of hypertension, although this is probably not so prevalent amongst the elderly. Both should indicate the need for careful control of the underlying condition, and in the case of diabetic retinopathy, xenon arc or laser coagulation are occasionally used. Macular degeneration, typically appearing as a coarse dark mottling in the macular area, has no specific treatment; but it is worth recommending the use of a magnifying glass for reading, and/or strong reading glasses. Often, however, patients will have discovered this for themselves.

Chronic glaucoma Chronic glaucoma can also lead to loss of vision and can either be the result of open-angle glaucoma, i.e. raised intraocular pressure unassociated with obstruction to the filtration angle of the iris, or a chronic form of the closed-angle variety. Until the visual loss is noted by the patient, these conditions may remain asymptomatic, and the prolonged rise in pressure will lead to a visual field defect and a pathological degree of cupping of the optic disc. This of course needs hospital referral when suspected, for supervision of medical treatment and consideration of drainage surgery if necessary.

It can be seen that careful examination of the eye is as important in the more chronic type of visual deterioration as it is in the case of acute loss of vision. It is also necessary to remember that in an old person more than one pathology may be responsible for the deficit. Since sight, together with preservation of mobility and intellectual capacity, is one of the major bastions of independence, it is extremely important to take seriously any complaint by a patient of loss of vision. In addition, since this section has attempted to cover only a few common situations arising in older people, the reader is referred to standard ophthalmological texts and to the need for specialist advice should the situation warrant it.

Blindness and mental health

There is evidence that blindness can affect mental health in old age. The following symptoms may develop as a result of blindness:

- Anxiety
- Depression
- Confusion, which usually results from isolation, but sensory deprivation can cause confusion even if the older person is not isolated.

These are not inevitable consequences of blindness, but develop if the old person and his relatives are not helped to adjust to the loss of vision.

Help for blind and partially sighted people

Because of the low expectations of elderly people and their relatives many older patients with visual impairment do not receive sufficient help. It is often assumed that nothing can be done to treat the cause of the visual problem or to investigate its effects. In addition for many elderly people their visual problem is not the most significant. One survey found that only 56 per cent of visually impaired old people counted poor sight among their greatest troubles. It has been estimated that the Blind Register only contains the names of two-thirds of blind elderly people, although 90 per cent of them are in contact with their general practitioner.

Registration is important because it brings some practical benefits, but the main benefit is that it brings the old person into contact with the social worker for the blind, who is able to advise the older person and his relatives. The social worker for the blind is based either in the eye hospital or in the social services department, and works closely with two new types of professional worker:

- The mobility officer, who is trained to help a blind person regain the ability to move about outside his home in confidence and safety.
- The rehabilitation officer, who helps the blind person regain the ability to look after himself and his home.

Unfortunately there are very few of these workers, so much of the support is left to the relatives of the blind person. There are a number of important points to emphasize to relatives:

- Help the old person make the most of the vision he has by keeping his spectacles clear and by ensuring regular checks at the optician's if he is not attending a hospital clinic. If ordinary spectacles are a problem the hospital clinic will be able to advise on low-vision aids such as magnifying glasses.
- Improve domestic lighting by putting in more powerful bulbs and moving lights closer to where the old person sits and reads.
- Try to encourage mental stimulation by arranging for volunteers to bring large-print books or cassettes from the library. The telephone and radio also offer very useful stimulation. The social worker for the blind will be able to advise about the telephones for the blind and radios from the blind charities.
- Try to prevent isolation if the old person lives alone by encouraging him to go out. The social worker or mobility officer should be consulted if isolation appears to be developing. Adjustment to blindness may be helped by attending a club run specially for blind people.

In addition relatives also need advice on two other important aspects of blindness—communication and mobility:

Useful advice for relatives on communication

Always let a blind person know when you are approaching.
Introduce yourself every time.
Hold his hand if he finds it helps him locate the position of your face.
Remember that blind people lose a great deal of what is going on by missing non-verbal cues, notably when they wish to enter a conversation. More formal verbal cues such as a question which includes the blind person, name etc., are therefore necessary. When a number of people are present the old person can be told to raise his hand if he finds it difficult to break in.
Always announce that you are leaving clearly and leave quickly after saying good-bye.

Useful advice for elderly patients and their relatives

Mobility

---

1 When guiding a blind person let him take your arm; do not grab him and try to steer him.
2 Let the blind person walk a little way behind you, about half a pace or so; do not push him in front. Tell him about obstacles before you reach them.
3 Always approach steps and kerbs at right angles.
4 To help him enter a car, place one hand on the roof above the open door and the other on the top of the door. When helping him to sit down do not try to reverse him into the chair; put his hand on the back of the chair and let him find his own way.

If the old person or his relatives are having difficulty, the mobility officer or social worker for the blind should be able to help.

Weight loss

Many elderly people seem to lose weight without passing comment on this fact. Consistent weight loss, however, is a symptom of significance and should always be treated seriously. Unfortunately, it is a common facet of so many conditions that the aetiology is often difficult to unravel. As is usually the case, it is best to start with a history and examination, since these will often indicate the most likely areas to pursue in more detail, although this is not always so, and it is then necessary to tackle the problems step by step. The outline below covers the majority of the important causes of weight loss. Malnutrition is a common factor causing or contributing to weight loss in the elderly and is discussed on page 111. Malabsorption, occurring less frequently, also requires consideration (p. 111). The other major causes of weight loss are described below.

Malignant disease of GI tract

A past history of pernicious anaemia, atrophic gastritis, or gastric ulceration indicates that the patient has a higher chance of developing a gastric carcinoma. This is a relatively common tumour in older people, and weight loss is often the only symptom. Quite advanced neoplasms can present with little more than weight loss and a mild degree of anaemia. Unfortunately, the majority of patients with this condition are suffering with advanced disease by the time they present, even though the symptoms and signs are so minimal. Major surgery is rarely undertaken, but palliative operative measures can significantly improve the quality of life in an elder with an advanced growth if they are suffering from uncomfortable symptoms. In the majority of cases the diagnosis will be confirmed by barium meal or endoscopy.

If the weight loss is accompanied by dysphagia, a malignancy in the oesophagus must be considered, although a carcinoma in the fundus of the stomach or indeed a benign stricture at the bottom of the oesophagus are also important causes. The investigations are the same as for a suspected carcinoma of the stomach.

Weight loss associated with rectal bleeding, or a disturbance of bowel function, should be treated in the same way in an older person as in a younger patient, namely with a sigmoidoscopy and barium enema. It is important not to assume that these symptoms indicate a definite neoplasm and that age is a contraindication for surgery. The elderly are of course prone to the same non-malignant conditions which cause this symptomatology in young people, for which treatment can be very rewarding.

Peptic ulceration   A chronic peptic ulcer often leads to weight loss. The same measures are adopted in older people as in their younger counterparts when dealing with peptic ulcers.

It is also very important to remember that a gastric ulcer which does not heal after an adequate trial of therapy should be biopsied in case it is malignant.

Carcinoma of the pancreas   This neoplasm is common in the elderly and is often found to be the cause of a painless obstructive jaundice. It may, however, present as weight loss, with little else to indicate its presence. It is then very difficult to diagnose and not infrequently remains unsuspected until further symptoms develop. A carcinoma of the head of the pancreas is often associated with epigastric pain, which characteristically often radiates into the back and may be relieved by leaning forward. This is a very difficult neoplasm to remove surgically, but if obstruction to the biliary tree results, a patient's quality of life can often be considerably improved with the help of palliative surgery, such as a by-pass procedure. This may change a miserable outlook to one in which the patient can live a meaningful existence for several months before he dies. If this condition is suspected it is probably best to refer the patient to a surgical or gastroenterological outpatient department for further investigation.

Endocrine conditions

Although diabetes mellitus and thyrotoxicosis can both cause weight loss in older people, thyrotoxicosis is the less common of the two and often presents in an atypical manner. Diabetes should of course be suspected if there is a history of increasing thirst and polyuria, often most strikingly manifested as nocturia, as well as weight loss. Often, however, the symptoms are not volunteered, or are misrepresented in such a way that they are considered to be indicative of another pathology, for instance a urinary tract infection. The symptoms are very similar to those in younger people, although more frequently than in the latter the patient presents in coma or pre-coma, since so many elderly people live on their own with nobody to report their illness, or urge them to seek further attention. Thyrotoxicosis can present as an apathetic patient with atrial fibrillation, a goitre, and weight loss, rather than the more typical presentation with hyperactivity seen in younger people. The diagnosis of both these conditions and their management is along the same lines as in younger people, and treatment is further discussed elsewhere (diabetes, p. 70; thyrotoxicosis, p. 128).

Psychiatric disease

Depression can present with weight loss and is easy to miss. When diagnosed it must be remembered that many of the drugs normally prescribed are likely to precipitate side-effects in older people. If treatment is difficult or unsatisfactory, the patient should be referred for a psychogeriatric opinion. Where appropriate, it is often more satisfactory for the patient to undergo a course of ECT than a prolonged course of antidepressants.

The other common psychiatric cause of weight loss is dementia. Senile dementia is considered at length elsewhere (p. 66), but unless there is a treatable cause for the intellectual deterioration, there is little that can or should be done about the weight loss of terminal dementia.

Other conditions

A malignancy anywhere may cause weight loss. Other common tumours in addition to those already mentioned include bronchus, breast, lymphomas, and leukaemias. If a neoplasm is suspected it is best to attempt to define only those that may be treatable or open to the possibility of amelioration. An extensive and exhaustive hunt for a primary malignancy should not be undertaken in an older patient unless there is a good cause.

Cryptic infection is not an uncommon cause of illness discovered at post-mortem. In particular, the elderly are subject to subacute bacterial endocarditis and tuberculosis, both of which may present in a variety of ways and may not be discovered until after the patient has died. Although the investigations are the same as in a patient of a younger age, a very high index of suspicion is needed in the elderly, since these conditions and other cryptic infections often respond well to treatment.

Drugs as a cause of weight loss resulting from malabsorption have already been mentioned. Many other drugs, however, can also produce weight loss, for instance by causing anorexia. One of the commonest is digoxin, which should always be prescribed with caution, with the need for continued therapy reviewed from time to time.

A systematic approach to the problem of weight loss will often result in the elucidation of the underlying disease. In many instances, hospital referral is unnecessary for either investigation or management.

Weight loss check-list

Could the cause of the weight loss be:

1 Deficient intake (see p. 111)
2 Dental problems?
3 Dysphagia?
4 Malabsorption?
5 Peptic ulceration?
6 Neoplasm of stomach; large bowel; pancreas; elsewhere?
7 Diabetes?
8 Thyrotoxicosis?
9 Tuberculosis or other chronic infection?
10 Depression?

8 Prescribing for the elderly

The principles of prescribing for the elderly are similar to those in younger patients. The principal questions are: is the drug required at all and if so is this the right preparation in the correct dose; are the side-effects going to be worse than the therapeutic benefits; is this the best type of preparation (e.g. liquid versus capsule) and can the old person read the label and instructions easily; how am I going to check compliance; and probably most importantly, when am I going to review the need to continue prescribing this drug? Although these questions are similar in all ages there are many details which are different and extremely important to bear in mind at all times when prescribing for older people. Some of the more important are discussed below.

Older people are more susceptible to adverse reactions and one has to strike the balance between morbidity from side-effects and a therapeutic gain. This is particularly so in some drugs where the margin between therapeutic benefit and the problems of toxicity is very narrow, e.g. in the treatment of cardiological and neurological conditions such as cardiac failure and parkinsonism.

It is best if, where practical, one doctor is primarily responsible for all the prescribing for an individual elderly patient. In this way some of the hazards of polypharmacy may be avoided. In one study (Williamson 1978) it was discovered that 80 per cent of those admitted to geriatric wards were receiving drug treatment of one sort or another and 25 per cent of patients over 75 years old were receiving three or more drugs on a regular basis. Having one doctor principally involved in prescribing for each patient may also avoid the risk of repeat prescriptions being signed without adequate review of the need to do so.

Much new information on prescribing in the elderly is now available in England from the Prescription Pricing Authority (PPA). It is not surprising to learn that there has been a 17 per cent increase in items dispensed between 1977 and 1988, or that net ingredient costs have also risen by 44 per cent in real terms. What is totally unexpected is that prescriptions for those of pensionable age accounted for 96 per cent of the overall increase in prescription items (Griffin and Chew 1990). As a result, their share of the total prescriptions dispensed rose from 32 per cent to 41 per cent, corresponding to a rise from about 12 items per elderly person per year in 1977 to more than 16 items in 1988. By contrast, prescriptions to people below pensionable age remains almost unchanged at about 5.3 items per person per year.

What about very elderly people? The gross NHS expenditure is £1186 per year per patient over 75 years old (*versus* £178 for every person aged 16–64 years and £521 for those aged 65–74 years). Using estimations of prescribing frequency based on consultation rates, it has been estimated that the average number of prescription items per very elderly persons, per year rose from 17 per cent to 24 per cent from 1977 to 1988. The over 75s account for about 55 per cent of all prescriptions written for those of pensionable age, whereas this very elderly group only constitutes 44 per cent of all those over the age of 65 years. In summary, these figures mean that looking after old people is a very expensive business: you can look after more than six young people for the price of looking after one very elderly person for a given length of time.

Compliance

The study of compliance rightly, albeit belatedly, has been one of the growth areas of modern medicine. Four factors are generally agreed to be associated with good compliance and a low rate of problems:

The simplicity of the regime.
The absence of side-effects or the need to change one's life-style.
Clear and appropriate information.
The quality of the doctor–patient relationship.

Simple regimes

A simple regime contains as few drugs as possible in the simplest regime possible for the shortest time possible. This cardinal rule is the reason why we are right to reject the advice of the pharmacological purists who generally insist (e.g. in the columns of journals such as the *Drug and Therapeutic Bulletin*) that tablets containing more than one drug are to be eschewed because it is not possible to change the dose of each constituent in-dependently. Thus we should all be prescribing potassium supplements independently of diuretics. The danger here is that this may more than double the number of tablets the patient has to take. We have had instances where the patient has felt ill, and so stopped the potassium but carried on with the diuretic—and *vice versa*—with disastrous consequences. So it is important to distinguish polypharmacy (which is often unavoidable) from regimes demanding an unnecessary variety of pills.

How can unavoidably difficult regimes be made easier? One trick is for a relative to label an egg-box or ice-cube box with times and days of the week—so that the old person takes all the pills in one compartment at each specified time. This gets round the problem of unopenable containers, and the problem of forgetful patients not being able to remember if they have taken a tablet or not (whereupon some of our patients have taken more pills 'just to be sure'—only to forget this second dose an hour later and take a third dose). Calendar packs are another aid to forgetful patients—except that if they are forgetful, they are likely to misplace packs and start a new one, and then stumble on the first pack, and mistakenly think that they have missed a dose.

These difficulties are delineated to demonstrate the descent into chaos and randomness which so often afflicts prescriptions of the highest clarity. Rather than pretend that everything is ordered, we might do well to acknowledge to the patient that it is rare for tablets to be taken as prescribed, and to ask if they have any difficulties or comments. Patients are very considerate—and hate to shatter our illusions. We only realized this when we bought a machine for 'instant' measuring of drug levels. We check compliance before taking the blood sample and patients offer us their cosy lies—but when they see that they are about to be confronted with a drug level the real truth finally comes out—in the words of one patient 'Well, actually, doctor, I usually *do* take these pills as you suggest, but I haven't taken any since I had the 'flu: you don't mind, do you?'

Adverse effects of treatment

If treatment has adverse effects on the patient, either drug side-effects or a major change in life-style, the probability that compliance will be poor is increased. Some treatments inevitably involve side-effects or change in life-style, but every effort should be made to minimize them. The need for careful follow-up is obvious and widely appreciated, but many problems still occur because insufficient attention is paid to the review of long-term medication. This is not to argue that repeat prescriptions should never be issued without seeing the patient; but it is necessary to work out a system which allows for the review of elderly people on long-term medication at a frequency which is convenient and appropriate to each case.

Clear and appropriate information

The instructions given to the patient should obviously be clear. They should obviously be set in words and terms familiar to the old person and if written instructions are given they should be printed in type big enough for the old person to be able to read it—typewriter capitals are a good size, and lines should be double-spaced. It is, however, also important that the information is appropriate to the patient's beliefs about his disease and treatment.

The incorporation of the patient's beliefs about disease and treatment into his education has been called the 'health belief' approach and it has been shown to be effective in influencing patients and improving compliance. The beliefs that must be taken into account when educating a patient are his belief about:

(a) the seriousness of the disease 'Does it cause serious disability or only minor inconvenience?'
(b) his personal susceptibility to the unpleasant consequences of the disease: 'Is it a one in a million or one in ten chance that I could be seriously affected?'
(c) the benefits of therapy: 'Will the treatment work, or am I too old for treatment?'

Advice has therefore to be based not only on pharmacological evidence but on the patient's own beliefs and attitudes, and, as we have already emphasized, these are particularly important when treating older people because many older people assume that they are suffering from the effects of ageing, which they know to be inevitable and untreatable, when they are in effect suffering from the effects of a treatable disease.

The doctor–patient relationship

Because of the scientific rigour of modern professors and editors and those who dispense research funds most research workers focus on those aspects of medicine which can be measured, counted, and chi-squared. Valuable though this approach has been, it has meant that those aspects of medicine which did not lend themselves to measurement, counting, or statistics have been relatively ignored, and one of these is the quality of the doctor–patient relationship. There is good evidence that the quality of the relationship is an important determinant of good compliance, and of course general practitioners have, in general, a good relationship with their elderly patients. Because of this, Dr James Knox argued in a very useful review of prescribing for the elderly in general practice that the magnitude of the problems had been overestimated because many of the studies had been hospital based. The doctor who is interested in his patient's beliefs and sensitive to his fears will achieve better compliance than the doctor who is, or appears to be, less interested.

Pharmacokinetics and pharmacodynamics

Pharmacokinetics and pharmacodynamics differ in older patients and this will have a bearing on the dosage of many drugs. Factors such as the different distribution of drugs within different body compartments, impaired metabolism, and renal clearance and altered sensitivity to some drugs, e.g. an increase in sensitivity to nitrazepam and a decrease for beta-blockers, further complicate the issue. In general where there is any doubt it is better to err on the side of giving too low a dose.

Drug interactions

The elderly are more prone to drug interactions than are younger people in whom usually a single disease is being treated. The coexistence of multiple pathologies, especially in those aged 70 and over, makes it much more likely that they will be taking a range of therapeutic agents. The interactions which may occur are legion, but most easily considered in terms of the site at which the interaction occurs. Some examples are as follows:

- **Drug absorption**   Drugs that have anticholinergic properties not only cause constipation but may also decrease gastrointestinal motility and either increase or retard the absorption of drugs, depending upon whether they are absorbed from the stomach or lower down the gastrointestinal tract.
- **Protein binding**   Many drugs are transported in the bloodstream bound to carrier proteins. Interference with anticoagulation is well known, e.g. salicylates increasing the effect of warfarin by displacing it from its binding sites; but there are many other examples. It is therefore important to take this into account if patients appear to develop side-effects after their therapeutic regime has been altered. Some of the commoner drug interactions are listed as an appendix in the back of the *British National Formulary*.
- **Hepatic enzyme induction**   Some medications, e.g. phenytoin, can induce liver enzymes which in turn affect the metabolism of vitamin D such that the patient is at an increased risk of developing osteomalacia. A similar problem occurs with the use of barbiturates, but as these are now so rarely prescribed, even for older people, it occurs less frequently in this context. In general, drugs that affect liver enzymes and those that alter renal clearance are likely to have secondary effects on the way in which other therapeutic agents affect an elderly person.
- **Competitive binding at receptor sites**   This is particularly a problem with drugs that act on the CNS, either as their main target or as a side-effect. Phenothiazines for instance block the dopamine receptors in the striatum, which results in drug-induced parkinsonism. This will obviously not respond to prescribing levodopa preparations and is the reason that patients in whom the parkinsonism is slow to respond to withdrawal of a phenothiazine, or in whom the medication cannot be withdrawn, need to be prescribed an anticholinergic preparation. Another example is the anticholinergic effect of some antihistamines, which block some classes of cholinergic receptors.

Polypharmacy

One of the most important points to consider when prescribing for an older patient is when to review the benefit or otherwise that the patient is experiencing. Polypharmacy often originates simply because of a failure of the prescriber to consider discontinuing a course of treatment.

The remainder of this chapter will discuss some of the pitfalls and problems associated with some of the drugs prescribed for older people. It does not contain an exhaustive list of side-effects, and nor is it meant to, but is designed to bring to the attention of the reader problems which are commonly encountered and which should be considered before prescribing the preparation in question.

Hypnotics

Before prescribing a hypnotic it is important to be clear in one's mind why it is required, and to try alternative means of producing sleep before prescribing a drug. Sometimes the problem identified by the old person is not a problem which requires treatment. Some old people become anxious that they are not sleeping as well as they were without appreciating that their decreased levels of physical and mental activity and their daytime naps reduce the need for sleep at night. Sometimes the anxiety about sleeplessness becomes the main factor perpetuating the sleeplessness (Fig. 8.1, p. 146).

Useful advice for old people and their relatives

Preventing sleeping problems

The most important means of preventing or treating sleeping problems is to establish a pattern of behaviour which will be followed every evening, for example:

9.30 p.m.: A warm drink, such as *Horlicks*®, *Ovaltine*®, or cocoa, not tea or coffee, or an alcoholic night-cap if there are no contraindications. This should be taken sitting in the same chair, perhaps with music playing but no television after 9 p.m.

9.45 p.m.: Bath

10.15 p.m.: Read some soothing book or magazine, not a thriller.

10.30 p.m.: Go to a bed, which should be warm and well made.

10.45 p.m.: Lights out.

If the patient complains that this regime is unutterably boring—explain that this is the whole idea. An alternative to the above is a bout of sexual intercourse.

In trying to sleep better, the old person who is anxious about his sleeping may try a number of different approaches, and this in turn increases the problem because an established pre-sleep ritual is a very important means of promoting sleep, and the old person should be encouraged to try to re-establish a set sequence of events before he goes to bed before a hypnotic drug is prescribed.

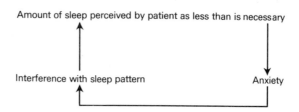

Fig. 8.1 The vicious cycle of insomnia.

Sleeplessness may be the result of remediable problems such as ischaemic limb pain, nocturia, orthopnoea, depression, etc. The hypnotic may be necessary in addition to treatment for another condition, and if so one must remember to discontinue the hypnotic when the underlying condition has been treated. The benzodiazepines are probably the most widely prescribed hypnotic, and the starting dose should be half that used in younger patients. Where possible it is probably best to use one of the shorter-acting drugs, e.g. triazolam (0.125 mg). If a benzodiazepine is inappropriate, chlormethiazole is a useful alternative—but may be addictive.

Tranquillizers

Tranquillizers may be used to lessen the level of agitation without making the patient drowsy. As with hypnotics it is important to discover why the patient is agitated in case the cause of the agitation also requires treatment. Phenothiazines of the chlorpromazine type should be avoided wherever possible and a small dose of a benzodiazepine, e.g. oxazepam or mild phenothiazine such as thioridazine tried instead. A small dose of haloperidol may be helpful, especially for maintenance treatment.

Whatever the dose of phenothiazine or haloperidol, side-effects such as parkinsonism, tardive dyskinesia, drowsiness, and postural hypotension must be watched for. In the case of phenothiazines especially, hypothermia and cholestatic jaundice may occur.

There are many potential contributory factors to anxiety, alleviation of which may obviate the need for drug treatment.

The principal cause of anxiety is uncertainty, and there are many uncertainties in old age. Some of the more common are:

Will I have to go and live in a home?
Will I develop dementia?
Will I become a burden on my family?
Will I fall again?
WIll I be incontinent again?
Will I be able to pay my fuel bills?
Will I be mugged?

These are only a few of the more common causes of anxiety. The old person may complain of anxiety, but the problem may present in other ways; or the patient may be referred by relatives without mention of anxiety. Anxiety may cause:

Weight loss.
Alcohol abuse.
Neglect of self or environment.
Agitation or restlessness, or confusion.
Preoccupation with physical symptoms.

Patients who are demented may also become anxious, and the management of anxiety is made more difficult if the person is unable to communicate why he is anxious. Anxiety is aggravated by isolation, because a small worry

---

Useful advice for old people and their relatives

Helping to control anxiety

1 No matter how trivial the matter seems take time to discuss it.
2 When listening look calm and confident and do not be afraid to hold the person's hand to reassure him while talking to him.
3 Do not just say 'Don't worry.'—take some positive step to reduce the cause of the anxiety, if the older person can identify a cause.
4 Suggest that the priest call, if the old person is religious. Prayer is often very helpful.
5 Try to reduce the old person's isolation.
6 Inform your general practitioner of the anxiety if it lasts for days, or if it intrudes into every thought or conversation, or if it is not allayed by solving the problem which the old person has identified as the cause of his anxiety.

can prey on the mind of an isolated person and assume a significance which is out of all proportion to the actual size of the problem.

Before prescribing a tranquillizer, it is appropriate to try and give simple advice to the elderly person and his relatives.

Diuretics

Loop diuretics, i.e. those acting on the loop of Henle, are usually unnecessary in older people as maintenance therapy for cardiac failure or hypertension. Milder diuretics are preferable, e.g. the thiazides. The loop diuretics most commonly used are frusemide and bumetanide. They can cause such a profound diuresis with alterations in plasma volume and plasma electrolyte levels that many patients experience severe side-effects, especially hypotension, as well as the social embarrassment of needing to make frequent visits to the toilet.

Potassium supplements are necessary in the majority of patients on diuretics, unless they are taking a potassium-sparing compound such as spironolactone, amiloride, or triamterene. It is not adequate to just measure the serum potassium level, since 200–300 mmol of potassium may be lost before there is any fall in a serum level. Plasma urea and electrolytes should probably be checked at least every six months in patients on long-term diuretic therapy. In many patients a soluble form of potassium is preferable to tablets.

It should be remembered that thiazides can aggravate or precipitate hyperuricaemia and diabetes, and that diuretics should rarely be prescribed for ankle oedema unless this is caused by heart failure.

Digoxin

Digoxin is rarely indicated in elderly patients in sinus rhythm. The major indication for prescribing it is the patient with atrial fibrillation and mitral valve disease. Very few patients need digoxin because of heart failure in other circumstances.

This drug is renally cleared from the body and therefore affected by the decreased renal clearance which is present in so many of our elders. Loading doses should never be more than 0.5 to 1.0 mg in divided doses over 24 hours, and in many patients a maintenance dose as little as 0.0625 mg will be sufficient.

In theory it is best to check on the following before prescribing digoxin: serum potassium and urea levels, an ECG to exclude conditions such as heart block, and ventricular dysrhythmias, including multiple ectopics.

Overdosage in the elderly is common and manifested by symptoms such as nausea, vomiting, anorexia, diarrhoea, confusion and disturbance of cardiac rhythm, as well as the more classical xanthopsia.

Antihypertensives

Many older people are unnecessarily treated for hypertension (see p. 86). If there is evidence of marked end-organ damage consider initiating treatment. It is probably still best to start with a diuretic, adding a beta-blocker if necessary, although some doctors prefer to use a vasodilator. If this approach is chosen it is particularly important to be aware of the sometimes catastrophic degree of hypotension or postural hypotension that an elderly person may develop. There are, in addition, the particular problems of ACE inhibitors, which are described later. Other drugs whch should be specifically avoided, if possible, are guanethidine, bethanidine, debrisoquine, reserpine, and methyldopa. Many of these are now no longer in use in UK practice. The usual precautions and side-effects that have to be considered when prescribing diuretics and beta-blockers must not be forgotten.

Drugs for parkinsonism

Until recently, L-dopa preparations were well accepted as the front line for treatment of Parkinson's disease. However, it is becoming common practice to withhold L-dopa until its use is warranted by the severity of functional disability. Apart from avoiding side-effects, the thought is that as L-dopa often only gives relief for a limited number of years, this is best held in reserve for when its use will be most appreciated in combating severe disease. In addition, evidence is accumulating that selegiline 10 mg/24 hours by mouth delays disease progression, making it appear to be an attractive agent to consider *before* the use of L-dopa. See p. 120.

Most of the drugs used to treat parkinsonism have a very narrow margin of safety between the therapeutic effect and toxic levels. Common side-effects include confusion and hypotension, and the anticholinergic properties of some of them may precipitate glaucoma and urinary retention.

Antimicrobials

From the general practice point of view the most important drug to use with caution is probably tetracycline and its derivatives. Tetracyclines can raise the blood urea in patients with impaired renal function, even to the extent of producing severe renal failure. These preparations are almost exclusively cleared from the body via the kidney, and one should at least have no reason to suppose that the patient has abnormal renal function before prescribing a tetracycline derivative.

The exception to this is doxycycline, which is mainly excreted through the bile and is therefore safe in the presence of renal failure. It has the added advantage of a single daily dosage compared to the t.d.s. or q.d.s. administration needed with the others.

Drugs for diabetes

Fortunately, few elderly patients require insulin, but when they do practical problems may make control of the plasma glucose level difficult. In particular, insulin is difficult to administer if the patients have arthritis in their hands or failing eyesight. The latter will also make it difficult for them to adequately assess the glycosuria they are producing. It may well be necessary to ask the district nurse or a relative to undertake this, and in most patients a once-daily injection regime will suffice, avoiding too large a burden on the person administering the insulin. Specially adapted syringes are available for the use of partially sighted diabetic patients. These rely on delivering a metered dose per push of the plunger.

When a drug is being prescribed for maturity-onset diabetes, most physicians use a sulphonylurea rather than a biguanide in the first instance. The short-acting sulphonylureas are preferable to the others such as chlorpropamide, since the long half-life of the latter coupled with its renal clearance has resulted in many instances of catastrophic hypoglycaemia. Sulphonylureas unfortunately make many patients feel hungry, and consequently they may have difficulty in sticking to their diet. Dietary treatment in the elderly is in itself often unsatisfactory because food is one of the few pleasures left to an older person; but weight reduction should be tried.

If a biguanide is added to the drug regime, metformin should be used (phenformin has been discontinued because of problems with lactic acidosis). Biguanides are best used in combination with a sulphonylurea and are rarely satisfactory on their own.

Antidepressants

See pages 69–70.

ACE inhibitors

The angiotensin-converting enzyme inhibitors (ACE inhibitors) are now becoming more widely used in older patients. It looks as if they may be particularly helpful in treating refractory cardiac failure, and the two preparations most frequently encountered at the time of writing are captopril and enalapril. Both of these drugs can cause a profound drop in blood pressure, and should initially be prescribed as a test dose. In the case of captopril the hypotensive effect is usually seen within one or two hours after the patient takes the tablet, but in the case of enalapril it is often delayed for six to eight hours and may also last longer than the hypotension caused by captopril. This hypotensive action is more likely to happen if the patient is already taking diuretic treatment and especially if he or she is hyponatraemic and/or hypovolaemic. When there is pre-existing renal impairment or the concomitant prescription of potassium-sparing diuretics, hyperkalaemia can also be a problem. The dose of both these preparations should therefore be reduced in the presence of renal impairment, and some authorities believe that treatment with an ACE inhibitor is best initiated in hospital, or at least where the patient can be carefully monitored. A cautious initial dose of enalapril is 2.5 mg and of captopril 6.25 mg. Captopril may be preferable in the elderly because of its shorter duration of action. The place of other ACE inhibitors in older patients has yet to be established, as at the time of writing they are only just beginning to be made available for general prescription.

9 Dying at home

The following ingredients (given in a suggested order of importance) are helpful in determining the success of terminal care given by GPs to patients in their own home (the question of what constitutes 'success' will be tackled in the last section of this chapter).

- A patient who trusts his or her doctor.
- Time to listen to the patient.
- A doctor who is sufficiently robust to withstand the pressures which so often accompany death at home.
- Leadership abilities.
- Relatives who can accept support and are not too easily exhausted.
- Flexible community-based nurses.
- Ready access to simple items of nursing equipment.
- Biological know-how, coupled with a good working knowledge of pharmacology.

These items will be explained in turn.

Trust

It has been said that where there is no trust there can be little healing, and no sharing of the process of illness—and what cannot be shared may prove to be unendurable. What is unendurable may manifest itself in the form of denial, anger, violence, and retreat into a negative world of self-pity. These are often normal reactions on hearing of one's terminal diagnosis. But with the availability of someone trusted (ideally, but not necessarily, the patient's own general practitioner) these negative emotions may be guided into a framework in which death is seen as natural, and something to be accepted.

There are no prospective trials of the usefulness of trust in helping the dying: but we must not ignore what we cannot measure. This is one reason why this item is the first on our list. Another reason is that if the doctor has tried to encourage trust and is consistently failing, he or she should consider enlisting the help of a colleague, who may meet with more success. We cannot be all things to all our patients. Rather than stumbling on in the darkness of trustless consultations we should allow someone else the chance to illuminate the therapeutic encounter.

But the most telling reason for putting trust first on the list is that without it none of the above ingredients of good terminal care may be achievable. So the doctor may arrange things, albeit subconsciously, so that as little time as possible is spent with the patient (e.g. visits arranged just before evening surgery)—or the nurse (or doctor) may be denied access to the house—or the drugs prescribed may be rejected.

Trust is a trick—and one where we very often do not know the mechanism. Nevertheless, the following analysis of a few of the mechanisms of trust may provide a helpful sketch.

Personal trust: To the casual observer, the doctor's bedside conversation about the patient's garden, or about the book he or she is reading may appear to be just small talk. But in reality, the doctor and his patient are like two people bargaining in an eastern bazaar: they are engaging in a process of mutual assessment. Once trust has been established, the sale (or, in this case, the therapeutic encounter) proceeds. This may be how trust is established; but how is it deepened?

Physical contact (e.g. the act of supporting a dying person or of feeling the distempered part) is one potent way of deepening trust. Another way is to correctly guess what the patient is thinking—particularly what he is fearing. In this regard, the dying patient's general practitioner will usually have a huge advantage over other professionals coming in to help: he or she will *already* know the patient and the family, and very often may be able to guess correctly what is uppermost in the patient's mind (the fear of pain, fear of a perceived after-life, fear for those dependants left behind).

Professional trust: In medical circles, it is often said wistfully that doctors are now not held in the high regard that was formerly the case. Patients are always questioning our diagnoses, questioning our motives and re-interpreting our prescriptions ('Ah!—MST: I know that. It's nothing but morphine. It's what they gave my sister when they polished her off. Made her sick as a dog. I'm not having any of that.'). However, it is very often the case that, when engaged in terminal care, these interrogative characteristics of our patients may be used to advantage. Rather than the doctor issuing edicts from on high, an interactive process can be established whereby the doctor explains all the options to the patient (hospice care, hospital care, pain clinic for out patient procedures, visiting Macmillan nurses, district nurses and general practitioners, slow-release tablets, four-hourly medicines, injections or other agents)—and the patients choose what they want, knowing that they can change their minds whenever they want. By putting the patient in charge there is the possibility of engendering a deepening trust beyond that which was fostered in 'traditional' medical interactions. The only problem is that one has to be more agile in anticipating what the patient wants.

One simple and practical way of engendering trust is to give your dying patient your home telephone number. Giving this information shows that you trust your patient, and the reciprocal result is the enlarging of your patient's trust for you (this rule of reciprocity is at the root of the 'trick' of trust-making referred to above). In our experience, this trust has never been abused—and it gives some patients and their relatives an enormous feeling of security to know that their very own doctor will be available at the moment of death. Critics will say that such actions as giving your home phone number encourages doctor-dependency. In reply to this criticism it must be acknowledged that doctor-dependency is very common in terminal care—and that it does not matter. Unlike the case in other therapeutic circumstances, where the doctor must have a weather-eye on the patient's future health-seeking behaviour, this consideration has no relevance in terminal care, because there will be no future circumstances in which the patient is going to suffer from any ill effects of doctor-dependency. This fact may be one explanation of why general practitioners enjoy their terminal care so much: they can give a fuller rein to their subconscious desires to dominate and be loved by their patient than is normally allowable in clinical practice.

Time to listen to the patient

A great deal can be done for the dying and their relatives within the confines and restrictions of the usual general practice day: that is, in surgeries and in home visits. The average time of consultations in general practice is from 5 to 10 minutes—and this fact is often cited to demonstrate what is said to be the inevitably superficial nature of GPs' contacts with their patients: 'perfunctory care by perfunctory men'. Is this picture accurate? The first thing to point out is that 5–10 minutes is only an average time. Much longer consultations can be arranged as needed—to compensate for those consultations which are very short (e.g. someone needing a certificate to be off work, or someone simply needing a blood-pressure check). Nevertheless, if the doctor works to a strict appointment system, he or she will often be aware of running late, and it is all too easy for the patient to pick up the GP's urgency to get through the consultation, and so keep his fears to himself. We are all aware of times when we have colluded with this state of affairs by subconsciously exhibiting our busyness to our patients to stem a tide of feelings which we do not want to hear in case they make us even later for the next appointment.

There are two ways round this problem. The first one that has been used is for the receptionist to ask the patient how long he or she needs for their appointment. On hearing of this novel idea, many will have imaginings about their most demanding patients insisting on appointments lasting the whole morning—and the immediate response is to declare that such a system is unworkable. In fact, this system has been observed closely, and there is no doubt that most patients choose an appropriate length for their consultations (Harrison 1988).

The second way around this problem is not to have an appointment system at all. Under this system, the doctor can never be late, as he has no times to keep to. The patients in the waiting-room have chosen to come and wait, and the doctor can simply get on with the problem in hand, devoting as much time as is required by the patient, without feeling that he is letting down his other patients. Some patients may have long waiting-times. Do they mind? The answer is that most patients are satisfied or very satisfied by whatever system their doctor adopts. In a recent patients' participation meeting to which the author was invited, one patient suggested (rather half-heartedly) that an appointment system should be introduced in a practice which did not have one (as a matter of policy). No patient supported this idea, and many commented vociferously that they valued the freedom of being allowed to turn up to surgery when they wanted.

On first looking at the problem, it might be thought that little terminal care will go on in ordinary surgery times, and that dying patients will normally be looked after at home. This, however, is not the full picture, and to accept it as such robs terminal care of a very valuable asset: the early preparation for accepting a fatal diagnosis. The message is: do not wait for the patient to become moribund, and in need of round-the-clock home care, before instituting the central precepts of terminal care. Terminally ill patients often have good days and bad, and if it is convenient for them, it may be suitable to ask the patient to pick a good day and come to see you in the surgery (this is easier to arrange if you do not have an appointment system). This is good for morale, as it is a manifestation that the patient can still engage in the activities of daily living. But it may deceive the doctor that the patient is getting on better than is, in fact, the case. For this reason alternating (and then more frequent) home visits by the doctor are suggested. So terminal care starts in the surgery, moves to the bedside—and then returns to the surgery as the bereaved do their grieving.

Home visits are an essential ingredient of terminal care, not least because they give unique insights into the patient's personality, and his or her hopes and fears seen in the setting of family life—compared with the more anonymous surroundings of the surgery. This is the reason why a few home visits early on may pay a disproportionate dividend later, and allow care in the surgery to be deeper, and to be grounded in a shared knowledge of family circumstances. On one memorable occasion, the author, not following his own rules, was called on a home visit to a very pleasant but notoriously neurotic lady with 'flu. As I was leaving she asked if I would like a word with her husband. On entering his bedroom, I was amazed to find a stoical old patient of mine with advanced lung cancer, whom I had been seeing in surgery frequently, and whom, for some reason, I thought was unmarried. So his wife's neuroticisms immediately became a little more understandable.

How is this shared knowledge of family life deepened? The first point to make is that there are no set rules: allow the patient to lead—and you follow wherever the patient takes you. Take as your starting point *whatever* the patient gives you. This may be verbal information—such as 'I'm sorry this room's in such a mess, but my grandson has just upset the Lego'—or non-verbal, such as photographs on a mantelpiece. In the latter case, and at a suitable juncture in the consultation, one can go further than simply enquiring as to who the people are in the photographs. If they are family members, you can ask, for example, who he/she takes after most: the patient or his/her spouse? In what way are they similar? In following up this train of questioning during succeeding visits ('Who will miss you most? your daughter or your husband?'), it is possible to build up quite an accurate picture of the patient's emotional life, without your own precepts intruding. (This method of questioning is the central insight of the discipline known as the psychology of personal constructs.)

How long should home visits be? When caring for the terminally ill, it is wrong to believe that only prolonged and detailed (almost morbid) consultations are all that are of value. The patient will not, in all likelihood, want to spend hours discussing his or her death at every consultation. The aim is to make oneself available—e.g. by 'popping in' frequently—just to let the patient and their family know that you are ready to discuss these things when the time is right: and to stop discussing them when there is no more to say (not simply when it is merely uncomfortable to say more).

To adopt the foregoing may not seem to have much to do with listening. But it is important in setting the tone for what can be called strategic listening: listening not to the idle prattle which can come to fill unheeding consultations, but rather to those central messages, sent consciously and unconsciously by your patient, and which reveal his inner world of hopes and fears. As a result of this listening your doctor may come to know more significant things about his patient than his closest friend or relative, so enabling him to make a unique contribution to the patient's welfare.

All the above can take place in the day-to-day life of general practice. No special arrangements need to be made. If extra time is to be spent with the dying, it must be taken from some other activity, as the general practice day is not infinitely expandable. The effective management of the primary health care team is important in allowing for this. If a job can be delegated satisfactorily, delegate it—to leave yourself with more time for those things that *only* you can do. Running through the heart of UK general practice is a fierce streak of independence. We are independent contractors, rather than being simply employed by health authorities; each GP is, to a large extent, a law unto himself, and he is not responsible to anyone for the decisions he takes; it takes, usually, an Act of Parliament to limit his freedom of action, there being no one else around to tell him what he can and cannot do; we like to do everything for our patients ourselves. This streak of independence in general practice is normally very healthy (and is partly responsible for the buoyant morale of GPs compared with colleagues in hospital), provided it does not make us too autocratic. However it does make us less good, perhaps, at working in teams. Rather than delegate we have tended to do everything ourselves (p. 177). This has sometimes led to ineffective use (at least in our own practice) of the skills in the primary health care team. By delegating more (e.g. blood-pressure checks, health 'MOTs', routine antenatal care, and follow-up of diabetic patients to properly trained practice nurses, nurse practitioners, and midwives) the doctor can be freer to engage in those activities at which he is most effective. Of course, the GP may find he is not very good at terminal care—so this itself may be what he delegates (his practice nurse may have a special skill in this regard), so that he can do something else particularly well (e.g. antenatal care, or care of diabetics). We can all ask ourselves the questions: 'What am I doing well that I could do even better if I had more time? What are the particular skills of the practice team? Am I using these most effectively?. What else could be safely delegated?' By answering these questions we can restructure the content of our working day, to allow *all* the talent in the practice to be effectively used.

A doctor who is sufficiently robust to withstand the pressures which often accompany death at home

It is of no use to the dying patient to have a general practitioner who is so sensitive as to render him impotent in the face of great grief. The patient does not want to be preoccupied by thinking up ways to comfort his doctor. It is not the case that we should never shed a tear with our patients: there is a time for this—but it is not all the time. To be of practical help we must channel the reawakening of our own griefs into energetic schemes of continuing care for our patient and his family, without being weighed down ourselves by the sorrow of the situation. One of the central dilemmas of terminal care is that if we disobey this rule, we become useless, whereas if we obey it in too muscular a way we stand to lose the very thing which is of most value in terminal care: namely sympathy. Too much sublimation of our own instincts will turn us into automata wielding catheter, syringe, and enema with a false compassion. We start out our medical lives strong on sympathy (and proportionately vulnerable in our own sensibilities) and weak on knowledge of the pharmacological basis of terminal care, and the danger is that this position is reversed—so that we become weak on sympathy in order to protect our own sensibilities, filling the void left by our declining sympathy with nothing but technical know-how.

So the central question is: How can we recapture the natural human quality of sympathy without incurring damage to our own sensibilities and *without* overburdening our patients with our reactions to their own grief? One partial answer to this difficult question is to work less hard. The author was once lucky enough to work in a practice where one of the partners decided to halve his work load. He and his patients certainly enjoyed a second flowering of his natural sympathy. In this Indian summer of his sympathy he became in many ways the ideal physician: wise, old, full of equanimity, experience, and empathy. However, this route is not open to us all, and it may be wrong to suppose that one can move straight from being a medical student to being a grand old physician, without some intervening stages of development—not least because if the wise words of grand old physicians were to fall from the lips of the young they would lose something of their weight and power, at least for some patients. So, short of suggesting special ageing clinics, where young doctors can acquire bald patches and wrinkles, this way forward may not, in general, be appropriate.

Another partial answer lies in increasing patients' autonomy—and in stepping back from unnecessary decision-making on their behalf. This is not only desirable in its own right, but it also has an important spin-off: by offering our patients the widest possible choice, we create the sort of environment in which we are most likely to get to know our patients best—because we learn what motivates them. By knowing our patients in this way an important and obvious insight declares itself. No two patients are the same. It is in the recognition of individuality that the spontaneous development of sympathy flourishes. If you find yourself getting bored with the repetitiveness of terminal care, seeing your patients as sets of interchangeable problem lists, this is a sure sign that you have not found out very much about your patients and that sympathy may be about to run out.

Leadership abilities

This refers not only to leadership within the primary health care team (a role normally, but not exclusively held by the general practitioner)—but also to leadership of the patient and his or her family. In many ways this is the obverse to the patient autonomy which has been given so much pre-eminence in the foregoing paragraphs. As an example of this sort of leadership, consider the next stage in the real life example given above of the stoical old man with advanced lung cancer and a very pleasant but neurotic wife. Some months later, after various unsatisfactory visits to the pain clinic, I found him at home, stoical as ever, but exhausted and in great pain. His wife persisted in underplaying his symptoms, being unable to admit that the crutch on which she had always relied upon for support now needed her. His deepest distress lay in his recognition of the fact that his wife would be unable to manage after his death. For this reason he did not want, voluntarily, to take adequate doses of oral opiates: he felt he had a duty to stay 'in charge' at all times. This was a sort of stalemate in which nobody was benefiting. What is the appropriate response here: reflection, conjecture, and the detailed exploration of the psychodynamics of their marriage—or decisive intervention? I was moved by the simple tragedy of a man unable to accept pain-relief and of a wife unable to bring herself to think of his approaching death. What was needed was a clear signal that being in charge was an illusion that would shortly be unsupportable and that his death was inevitable, and life without him would have to be faced. I therefore suggested that injections of diamorphine were needed 'on medical grounds', and husband and wife willingly acquiesced with this. I summoned various sons and daughters from other parts of the country, and once they were assembled, and were aware of the support that their mother would need, I began regular injections of diamorphine, doubling the dose at each injection, to ensure a painless death. What separates this from euthanasia is the intention of the doctor. The primary intention is to make sure that the patient *and the family* feel no pain or mental anguish. Doubling the dose of diamorphine at each injection is a reliable way of achieving these ends.

This might be described as the active management of death—akin to the active management of labour, the central precept of which is that mothers will not be left in labour for days on end, and that active steps will be taken to deliver the baby as soon as a certain time in labour has elapsed. Unless one has the ability to lead a family in the active management of death, one can get oneself into the worst of all possible worlds, in which the dying person's pain is uncontrolled, the family is weaving a cocoon of illusions which seems to deny this, and the doctor becomes party to this collusion by incorrectly holding to the premise that, because he has offered the patient and his family a full range of options (which they have declined to make use of), he has discharged his duty satisfactorily. In these circumstances, where an inadequate dose of diamorphine is used, and the process of death pointlessly prolonged, the relatives are likely to become exhausted, and then, once death has occurred, they blame themselves for failing the patient in his hour of need—either because he had to be taken elsewhere for his death, or because, in their tiredness, the relatives lapsed into selfishness and recrimination.

The other aspect of leadership which is important is leadership of the primary health care team. This normally falls to the general practitioner (probably because he has the power to prescribe, rather than because his skills in this field are universally acknowledged to be pre-eminent). Rather than note down platitudes about leadership of the primary health care team, it is probably more informative to give real-life examples of failures of leadership, and the consequences to the dying patient of such failures.

Mr D. R. was dying of stomach cancer and was being visited regularly but separately by a nurse from the local hospice. He had been taking co-proxamol for osteoarthritis, and, for a while, he had no pain. As soon as his pain began to break through, the GP prescribed morphine sulphate tablets, 30 mg, one to be taken twice a day, explaining that they were morphine-based and a small step up from his previous tablets, and that they should be taken regularly, even if the patient was not in pain at the time the tablets were due to be taken. The nurse from the hospice arrived at the same time as the tablets, and commented to the patient that they were very strong, and that 10 mg tablets would be better. It then became very difficult to persuade the patient to take the tablets. He thought (erroneously) that there would be nothing left in hand for when the pain got really bad—and so decided not to take *any* pain relief, and this state of affairs lasted a full two weeks. The issue here is not about whether the doctor or the nurse was correct, but about the lines of communication between members of the primary health care team.

There are two possible solutions: one reinforces the primacy of the doctor's authority, while the other reflects a more team-based approach. Either there must be a strict rule that all changes to medication are mediated directly by the doctor and nobody else—or, before starting therapeutic initiatives, the members of the team agree to discuss these first, on the view that *anyone* can then mediate therapeutic changes (spouse, nurse, hospice, or doctor) once the necessary discussions have taken place.

The advantage of the second option is that it is more flexible, and that decisions can be enriched by input from a wider range of people. The leadership involved here is much more a question of setting up these channels of communication—rather than dominating them, once they are in existence.

Relatives who can accept support and are not too easily exhausted

So far in this chapter, the role of the relatives has been taken for granted. But what happens if the patient lives alone, or if the spouse is unhelpful (e.g. if the husband is an alcoholic—or is himself very frail)? First let us take the problem of the dying patient who lives alone. Let us assume that there are no helpful neighbours (so often, however, *not* the case) and that the reason why he is alone is that he is a cantankerous old man—who puts everyone's back up. He cannot be persuaded to go into a hospital, nursing home, or hospice. The first rule here is to stop trying to persuade him to do anything, and to accept him as he is, without threats, enticements, or posturings of any kind. These are all failed solutions, and the danger is that the atmosphere of failure is augmented by perpetually going over the same ground. One way forward is to *do* nothing: simply *be* with him—until he leads you in the direction in which he wants to go. This may be the only way of engendering trust, which is, as indicated above, the cornerstone of successful terminal care.

If everything fails, and particularly if the district nurses are becoming exhausted and demoralized by looking after the patient, consider transferring that patient to the care of another practice. You can explain the problems to the new practice, and indicate that you are not abandoning the patient, and would be happy to take the patient back after a specified number of weeks, if the new practice is equally baffled by the problem. Forcing a dying man to change his doctor may seem cruel, and we only suggest it when things have got to the stage where the patient's current doctor is not making any useful contribution. Changing doctors must be a way of helping the patient—not just a way of helping the doctor. Even dying men can learn, and asking a patient to change his doctor is a powerful message which may alter attitudes and behaviour. This ability to learn is one of the central tenets of terminal care: the process of accepting a terminal diagnosis through a number of *learned* phases (shock/numbness → denial → anger → grief → acceptance → longing). To be successful, changing doctors must be a way of initiating movement along this sequence.

In those instances where the relatives are unhelpful, or very frail, the problem is very different. These circumstances do not necessarily mean that the patient cannot be looked after at home. It simply means that a greater than usual burden will be placed on the primary health care team. Here the vital ingredient is the detailed assessment of the home circumstances by an experienced nursing sister. If she is confident that the team can cope (e.g. if augmented by volunteers or extra nursing input) it is then possible to go ahead. If the assessment is unfavourable, this must be communicated to the patient and his family so that alternative hospice or hospital care can be arranged.

Flexible community-based nurses

This may seem an obvious ingredient that needs no extra comment. However, a number of developments in the provision of nurses in the community has greatly increased the quality and quantity of nursing input that is available. Some health authorities have made the funding of community (district) nurses a high priority, and this has had the effect in our own practice, for example, of more than doubling the number of nurses available. There are also NHS twilight and night nurses available. This means that injections and full nursing care can be given at all times of the day and night. If we had to identify one organizational aspect which has been most influential in allowing us to give optimal terminal care to our patients, it would be this ready access to skilled nursing. It is also the aspect of care which is appreciated most readily by the patient and his family. This service is what allows a reality to be made of the often-expressed ideal of being able to die at home with dignity, and surrounded by the family. Nurses themselves also find this round-the-clock provision of care very rewarding. Not all areas within our own health authority have access to twilight and night nursing services: those practices within the system find that they are more attractive to existing and incoming nurses because they are able to offer a better quality of care.

Ready access to simple items of nursing equipment

Very often the one item of equipment needed in a hurry, and often at inconvenient times, is a commode. Other nursing items frequently needed are urine bottles, incontinence pads, catheters, and bolsters to enable the patient to be propped up comfortably in bed. Hospitals frequently have a Red Cross loans department for a wide range of equipment, and it is a good idea to familiarize oneself with what is available. Many of us think that these items of equipment are only available during normal office hours when the loan department is open. However, the hospital porter always has a key, and can put out an item of equipment for collection by relatives, nurse, or general practitioner. Commodes will fit into most cars—including minis.

Biological know-how, coupled with a good working knowledge of pharmacology

So far, in our list of the leading ingredients for successful terminal care, attention has only focused on the personal aspects of the carers, and the organizational aspects of care. It is right that these two areas are given pre-eminence. Too often it is assumed that what is needed is simply technical know-how and all the other aspects can be taken for granted. But without the appropriate personal attributes and organizational back-up, no amount of biological and technical know-how will help. By biological know-how is meant that quality which arises slowly in nurses and doctors as a result of continuous exposure to biological events, and which allows them to understand intuitively the mechanisms at work in unfolding biological sequences—so allowing the events along the pathway to be foretold, interpreted, and sometimes pre-empted. It is the medical equivalent of the 'green fingers' so highly prized in the horticultural world. It may be more of a question of instinctive flair—rather than something to be learned: but if it can be learned, it must be learned directly from patients—and not from books such as this. We will therefore say no more about biological know-how, and turn our attention to technical and pharmacological matters in the pursuit of symptom control.

Symptom control has probably been over-emphasized in the past, and has erroneously been used by hospices as the yardstick for measuring the success of terminal care. It is as if all symptoms are anathema, and as soon as they appear they must be abolished—completely and utterly. This view stems from the rather cloying definition of health put forward by the World Health Organization. This is that health is a state of complete physical, mental, and social well-being. This is the aim of those who give pre-eminence to symptom control. But what happens if we substitute another, more dynamic definition of health. Take, for example, that provided by Illich (1976): 'Health designates a process of adaptation—to changing environments, to growing up and ageing, to healing when damaged, to suffering, and to the peaceful expectation of death. Health embraces the future . . . and therefore includes anguish and the inner resources to live with it.' On this view, symptoms have meaning—and to insist, at all costs, in abolishing them is to deny at least some patients, a means of making sense of their world, and of growing in stature. It is *not* our intention to foist certain definitions of health on our patients. Our point is simply that we must be prepared to offer our patients a variety of viewpoints, and be flexible enough ourselves to work within the bounds of the definition which is chosen (consciously or, more often, unconsciously) by the patient. Those who choose to die at home often have an independent streak within themselves, and often put other values higher than symptom control. For example, they may willingly (and occasionally joyfully) suffer agonies in making a journey to pay their final respects to friends, family—or simply to a well-loved landscape.

Effecting symptom control—an alphabetical directory (Regnard 1986)

1 Agitation—try *diazepam* 10 mg suppositories▲ (e.g. 10 mg/8 h) if the patient cannot swallow. *Haloperidol* 5–10 mg orally also helps (the liquid is 2 mg/ml and is supplied with a pipette). *Methotrimeprazine* (a group 1 phenothiazine) is another alternative (25 mg/8 h PO/IM).
2 Anaerobic odours—*metronidazole* 400 mg/8 h PO or 500 mg suppositories▲ mitigates such odours from large tumours—as do charcoal dressings (*Actisorb®*). Masking attempts with aerosol perfumes usually make equally unpleasant compound smells.
3 Bladder haemorrhage—*alum irrigation solution 1 per cent* by catheter (Bullock 1985). This is much safer than formaldehyde irrigation.
4 Bone pain from metastases—*naproxen* 250–500 mg/8 h orally after food is helpful (consider *splinting joints* if this fails). Naproxen suspension is 125 mg/5 ml, and naproxen suppositories▲ (500 mg) are also available.
5 Coated tongue—*hydrogen peroxide 6 per cent* solution or *pineapple chunks* chewed, to release proteolytic enzymes, helps and are refreshing.
6 Depression—*amitriptyline* (25–50 mg at night, increasing up to 150 mg/ 24 h orally). Amitriptyline suspension is 10 mg/5 ml. Injections are 10 mg/ml.
7 Diarrhoea—*low residue diets* may be needed, e.g. after radiotherapy.
8 Distension accompanying ascites—*spironolactone* 100 mg/12 h with *bumetanide* 1 mg/24 h, both orally, may reduce associated symptoms.
9 Dry mouth—chewing *pineapple chunks* helps as they release proteolytic enzymes. Sucking *ice* or *butter* also helps.
10 Dysphagia makes pills useless, so use *suspensions* or *suppositories* (*marked* ▲ *in this table*) instead. Palliative radiotherapy or endoscopic laser treatment may improve dysphagia.
11 Euphoria can be induced (in some patients) by using *steroids*. *Dexamethasone* 4 mg/12–24 h orally is the most usual. Tablets are 2 mg (≈15 mg prednisolone) strength.
12 Fevers of malignancy—*naproxen* 250 mg/8 h after food is helpful (see 4 above).
13 Gastric irritation, e.g. associated with gastric carcinoma can be helped by H_2 *antagonists* (e.g. cimetidine 400 mg/12 h orally; the suspension is 200 mg/5 ml).
14 Gastric stasis related with vomiting—*metoclopramide* 10 mg/8 h orally or subcutaneously helps. The suspension is 5 mg/5 ml. Avoid with

concurrent opiates, as there is antagonism; so use *prochlorperazine* 5–10 mg/8 h orally or twice daily suppositories▲ (25 mg), or *domperidone* 30 mg suppositories▲ three times a day.

15 Headaches of raised intracranial pressure may be reduced by using *dexamethasone* 4 mg/12–24 h PO. See item 11.
16 Massive haemoptysis—use IV *diamorphine* to relieve all distress rapidly.
17 Nerve destruction pain—*amitriptyline* (see 6 above).
18 Nightmares can be helped by *haloperidol* 5–10 mg orally (the liquid is 2 mg/ml and is supplied with a pipette).
19 Noisy bronchial rattles are helped by *hyoscine hydrobromide* 0.4–0.8 mg SC/8 h or 0.3 mg sublingually.
20 Opiate-induced constipation is helped by *bisacodyl tablets* (5 mg), one or two at night—or in suppository▲ form (10 mg).
21 Pain—*diamorphine* oral suspension: 2 mg ≈ 3 mg morphine. SC: 1 mg diamorphine ≈ 1.5 mg morphine. Diamorphine is the best parenteral drug as it is soluble, so that very low volume (so painless) injections may be given—for almost all doses. Oxycodone 30 mg suppositories▲ (e.g. 30 mg/8 h, ≈30 mg morphine) can be used for pain when dysphagia and vomiting make pills useless, as can *buprenorphine sublingual* 0.2 mg/8 h, which is not a pure agonist, so 'ceiling' effects limit the benefit from increasing doses, compared to oxycodone.
22 Pleural pain can be given lasting relief with *intercostal nerve blocks*.
23 Pruritus of jaundice is helped by *cholestyramine* 4 g/6 h orally (1 h after any other drugs).
24 Rectal discharges (foul)—*betadine vaginal gel*®.
25 Resistant constipation—*enemas* are useful (e.g. Arachis oil).
26 Resistant pain—*nerve blocks* can be useful.
27 Stimulating appetite—*dexamethasone* 4 mg/12–24 h PO may help.
28 SVC obstruction—give *dexamethasone* 8 mg IV stat helps symptoms. Prompt radiotherapy may be appropriate.
29 Vaginal discharges (foul)—*betadine vaginal gel*®.
30 Vomiting—*cyclizine* 50–100 mg/4–8 h orally, PR▲, IM, or SC, or *haloperidol* (see 18 above) are useful. When vomiting makes pills useless try *prochlorperazine* 25 mg suppositories▲ (e.g. 25 mg/12 h).
31 Vomiting from upper GI obstruction is helped by *hyoscine hydrobromide* 0.4–0.8 mg SC/8 h or 0.3 mg sublingually.

Two cardinal points

1 List every symptom the patient has, and diagnose each individually.
2 Make a plan for each symptom's relief, and review progress frequently.

For example, the patient may have constipation from drugs, a dry mouth from poor fluid intake, and 3 sorts of pain—e.g. from an invasive cancer, from bony metastases, and from abdominal distension from ascites.

The best place to die: home or hospice?

This is a question which we often ask ourselves—and this is where we make our first error. This is not a question to ask ourselves—but a question to ask our patients. Our job is to be in a position to provide the pertinent details to enable the patient to choose. Thinkers on this issue have coined the phrase quality of death—and have even tried to measure this (Wallstone 1988). The measurement centres around symptom control—and the defects of this yardstick have already been laid bare in the paragraphs above. There is, however, a more fundamental problem with the idea 'quality of death'; the moment of death is always the same—and its only quality is its finality, an all or nothingness which is not capable of division or demarcation. It is the quality of *life*, not of death, which is at issue.

So let us rephrase our question: which is the best place to live: home or hospice? How do we put ourselves in a position to provide the pertinent details to enable the patient to make a choice when asked this question by a patient? The first thing is to find out what 'pertinent' means for the individual patient with whom you are dealing. For one patient the crucial factor may be having a hand to hold at the moment of death. For another it may be fear of pain. For another, it may be fear or loss of dignity, or loss of independence. The next question is whether we mind if the patient's decision is a rational one. Doctors are frequently nervous of the irrational, and often we do not rest until a patient has taken a decision rationally. Does it matter if our patients chose the place of their final days according to other criteria than strict rationality? Probably not, particularly if no one else is harmed. Does it matter if their decision is based on a delusion—e.g. that there is no escape, once inside the hospice's precincts; or that it is irresponsible to one's neighbours to die at home? If death is near, it may be unwise to try to disillusion the patient. When the author has tried to do this, he has only bred suspicion and the elaboration of further delusions. The message is simple: relax—and let the patient make his own choices on any criteria—even on no criteria at all.

Part III   Management issues and prevention

10 The scope for prevention

Prevention in the elderly is qualitatively different from prevention in younger people because what one is trying to prevent is (usually) different. One is generally not seeking to prolong life so much as to enrich its quality. For example, one could argue that a patient who has had a myocardial infarction and also has a high cholesterol who is 75 years old will be unlikely to benefit very much from a diet designed to reduce his cholesterol intake. To adopt such a diet may annul one of the patient's chief pleasures in life: his food. Even discussing the problem may make the patient feel guilty after each creamy meal, and, worse still, it may make him nervously anticipate his myocardial infarction, or even bring one on. A better intervention would be to encourage regular gentle exercise, such as walking or swimming, as this is likely to promote a general sense of well-being. If the patient insists on your doing something to lower the risk of myocardial infarction one could consider suggesting a minute dose of aspirin. This would have the advantage of not infringing the patient's life-style, and not making him doctor-dependent—because he can buy the aspirin from the chemist. This illustrates the four cardinal principles of prevention in the elderly:

- Preventive activities should increase the quality of life.
- Preventive activities must be agreed with the patient, and not foisted on him or her.
- Preventive activities must not induce doctor-dependency or ill-health behaviour.
- Preventive activities must be based on the results of well-conducted trials. (We know that post-MI complications are reduced by about 20 per cent by exercise programmes and by aspirin—in the above example.)

There are many spurious preventive activities in the elderly which are presented to general practitioners from various sources such as patients, relatives, drug manufacturers, nurses, health visitors, and government—and it is wise to furnish one's mind with a way of assessing possible preventive activities. The four principles outlined above are useful in this regard. In certain instances we may accept preventive activities which flout one or other principle, but if more than one principle is flouted we require very powerful additional arguments before public money and our own energies are spent.

Let us now consider the spectrum of preventive activities. Readers should know and be able to reject the distinction which divides prevention into primary, secondary, and tertiary prevention (they should know of this distinction because it is often referred to and even more often misunderstood, and they should be able to reject the distinction because it is counter-productive—as illustrated below).

Primary prevention

Primary prevention prevents a disease before it has started to happen. Vaccination against tetanus is a good example of a valuable exercise in primary prevention in the elderly—because most of the UK deaths from tetanus are in elderly patients. Polio vaccination in the elderly is not such a good example because old people are not dying of polio, and the vaccination can have side-effects (including the arrival of virulent strains of polio as a result of passage through the old person's gut). Another example is the removal of a healthy appendix during a sigmoid colectomy; or the provision of a light in a dark passage before elderly clients arrive.

Secondary prevention

This is the treating of disease or conditions before they have become overt or symptomatic. Examples are *carcinoma-in-situ* of the cervix, or small breast carinomas detected in the well-woman clinic or by mammography. Another example is post-exposure hepatitis B or rabies vaccination—or diets for people who are simply obese, or putting a nitrate under the tongue *before* starting to run for a bus, or filling a tooth, or using chloroquine for malaria prophylaxis.

Tertiary prevention

This is the prevention of the adverse consequences of diseases or conditions which are already symptomatic. Activities in the diabetic and antenatal clinics fall into this category, as do the wearing of spectacles, bereavement counselling, coronary artery bypass grafting, and the nailing down of stair carpets after a fall.

The trouble with the primary/secondary/tertiary distinction is threefold.

1 As illustrated above, the distinction groups together activities which are totally different and share no common ground whatsoever. There are no generalizations that only apply to one of these types of prevention which are not trivially entailed by their definition. For example, it is quite untrue to say that the best form of prevention is primary prevention. It might be very wasteful. It is equally untrue to say that tertiary prevention is a very complex matter, and beyond the scope of simple books.
2 Philosophically, the distinction is ridiculous—as demonstrated by considering the prevention of sea-sickness. If you take a certain tablet while on dry land, is this primary prevention? What if you are already feeling queasy as you hear the waves pound the harbour wall? What is being

prevented in this case? Is there any qualitative difference in the prevention here and that in a passenger on board who can tell by the motion of the ship (covert disease) that there will be a vomit-inducing swell out to sea? The answer here is 'Don't bother about primary/secondary/tertiary distinctions: take the tablet as soon as possible.' Even more muddling (for those who are trying to uphold the distinction) is to ask what is happening when the traveller takes his next tablet, six hours later, and now far out on a choppy sea. Suppose that the tablet is working quite well: he is only feeling moderately sick. What started out as primary prevention (perhaps) has now become tertiary prevention but the whole exercise still counts as one into primary prevention if it was started on dry land and there was no pre-travel nausea (or an exercise in secondary prevention if the pill was taken just as long before travel, but on board the docked ship)

What is being prevented when a pacemaker is inserted? If the answer is falls it might be primary prevention, because the patient may not yet have had one; if it is done to prevent repeated asystole it is tertiary prevention; if it is done in the light of bundle branch block and left axis deviation it is primary prevention.

3 It might seem uncharitable to throw out a distinction just because it is philosophically flawed. After all we are quite happy to use Newtonian mechanics to predict the movements of red cells and planets even though the system is internally faulty. We cherish it because it is useful. But we reject the primary/secondary/tertiary classification because it is so *useless*. No one calls himself a 'specialist in tertiary prevention'—nor do we learn about prevention in any sequential way. We have never come across practices which hold clinics for only primary prevention but in which *any* form of primary prevention is allowable. And we certainly do not wake up in the morning and say 'Today will be a good day for secondary prevention: where shall we start?'

A much more useful distinction is to group those preventive activities which you do as an *integral part* of the consultation, and those which are loosely tacked on to it for public health reasons and could easily be done by your nurse. A third group comprises those preventive activities which must be carried out in the patient's home (prevention and the home environment). Let us look at these in turn.

Preventive activities which are integral to the consultation

Here is a list of examples (which span the primary/secondary/tertiary divide):

- Giving asthmatic patients a supply of steroids to start whenever needed.
- Giving bronchitic patients a supply of antibiotics for the bathroom cupboard.

- Giving potassium with loop or thiazide diuretics.
- Debriding wounds.
- Giving aspirin in unstable angina, or after transient ischaemic attacks.
- Giving anticonvulsants to epileptic patients.
- Giving warfarin in atrial fibrillation associated with mitral stenosis.
- Arranging coronary artery bypass grafts.

The list is almost endless, and comprises much of clinical medicine—and needs no further comment here. We do these tasks without really thinking of them as 'Prevention'—and they are largely uncontroversial.

Public health and prevention

Into this category falls all screening activity. It is an important area for the population as a whole, but, for reasons described in the first paragraph of this chapter, it is of less importance in the elderly. For example, we know that mammography, blood-pressure measurement, and screening for cervical cancer are not cost-effective in this group.

More cost-effective might be screening for glycosuria (the patient is likely to feel better as well as live longer if you detect his diabetes), glaucoma (in first-degree relatives of these with this condition), and deafness (p. 000).

Unreported health problems   A useful screening questionnaire to send to patients is known as the Woodside 9-item screening letter:

1 Do you live on your own?
2 Are you without a relative you could call on for help?
3 Do you depend on someone for help?
4 Are there many days when you are unable to have a hot meal?
5 Are you confined to home through ill health?
6 Is there anything about your health causing you concern or difficulty?
7 Do you have difficulty with vision?
8 Do you have any difficulty with hearing?
9 Have you been in hospital during the past year?

If a patient answers 'Yes' to any question, or fails to return the questionnaire, they are given a comprehensive assessment.

Because old people may not appreciate that a problem has developed, it is also worth while to consider asking:

'Have you developed any new health problem in the last six months?'
'Is there anything you cannot do now which you could do six months ago?'
'Are there any other problems that we can help you with?'

For further discussion, see Occasional Paper No. 35 published by the Royal College of General Practitioners entitled *Preventive Care of the Elderly: a review of current developments*.

In the UK, screening for undeclared health needs in the elderly is becoming ever more fashionable, to the extent that the Government has made annual visits from the GP to his elderly ($\geqslant 75$ yrs) patients a terms-of-service requirement (or, at least, an invitation to visit the patient's own home). Topics to be covered comprise:

- Annual home visit to see the home environment and to find out whether carers and relatives are available.
- Social assessment (life-style, relationships).
- Mobility assessment.
- Mental assessment.
- Assessment of the senses (hearing and vision).
- Assessment of continence.
- General functional assessment.
- Review of medication.

Practice management

Each British General Practice will find its own way to meet these requirements. Many are taking on extra practice nurses specifically for visiting the elderly at home, and most UK general practices either have a computer for call and recall purposes or have specific plans to purchase one. Both computers and practice nurses are expensive, with many hidden costs, and we cannot overemphasize (in the light of our own mistakes) how important it is to cost out each new initiative. For example, many of the GPs now employing practice nurses may mistakenly believe that they will always be reimbursed 70 per cent of their wages if they have been appointed before April 1990. It should be pointed out that FHSAs can change this if the nurse's hours are changed. In this case the GP might have to pay far more for his or her nurse than can be recouped through capitation allowances—or be involved in lengthy and expensive redundancy arrangements.

Community (district) nurses who are visiting patients anyway (e.g. for leg ulcers) will often be prepared to carry out the health check (and indeed will have already done most of it in their initial assessment). This may extend to the patient's spouse or other elderly people living in the same accommodation—but if it is to stretch beyond this, the GP would have to pay the nursing authority. The same would be true if the GP were to consider asking a health visitor (the most ideally trained candidate) to do the assessment.

The cheapest and most cost-efficient way of communicating with patients is to use the opportunity presented when they receive a prescription (either a repeat, or during a surgery consultation). An invitation to ask for a home visit can be slipped in with the prescription for the patient to read (or throw away) at his or her leisure. These letters can either be printed out separately, or, for computerized prescriptions on continuous stationery, they may occupy the very conveniently blank right-hand half of the prescription. It is an easy matter for a receptionist to put a month's worth of prescriptions through a printer so that the reverse side of the blank portion carries the letter, leaving the front side available for anything else the doctor wants to use it for (such as the patient's health check card, or other details). Some computers allow for keyboard customization so that at the press of a single pre-programmed key after each prescription the fact that an invitation has been sent to the patient can be recorded (along with the date, and the due date for one year's time, when, if the patient has not been issued with another prescription-cum-invitation one should be sent through the post). Careful reading of the keyboard manual can pay rich dividends in saving time and key-strokes. Ninety per cent of elderly patients will have had such invitations by the end of a year (many will have had six or more)—so the postal bill should not be too big. If it *does* seem rather big the computer can group patients according to street, so that invitations can be delivered *en bloc*, one street at a time, by a receptionist. It is not necessary to be computerized to have this facility. Some very well-organized practices keep an up-to-date street register of all their patients. This arrangement (either using a computer or a street register) will be less appropriate for very scattered rural practices. At the end of the month there will be many unused letters (those from prescriptions for those less than 75 years old), and these may then be used in following months, until the receptionist again needs to print out another batch. In our own practice we have so far issued over 300, letters and have had two positive responses. This low uptake on the general front stops us from being swamped and will allow us to target our preventive activities more accurately to those who are most likely to be in need, and most likely to gain real benefit.

Just how cost-effective is non-targeted care likely to be? The most recent evidence is that it will cost about $\geqslant £425$ per problem identified (Coleman 1989). This might be acceptable if the problems were major ones. In fact, among the 900 elderly Solihull patients screened (from a list size of 11 000), the yield was only four ameliorable problems—chiropody (1), meals on wheels (1), home aids (1), and optical (1). Two patients were found to have hypertension, but, as has been explained elsewhere (p. 86), this is not something one should either look for, or treat. The other very significant finding was that 51 per cent of the patients refused to be screened. Although the population invited may not be typical, this nevertheless gives rise to the idea that these patients' longevity may have something to do with their perception of themselves as being healthy and independent and able to stand on their own two feet. It is our hope that widespread screening will not transform these sterling characters into doctor-dependent patients. Earlier trials have also suggested that screening of the elderly is not a very cost-effective pastime (Stringfellow 1987), although other earlier studies from

Denmark and Wales have shown that those screened were admitted to hospital less often, that they felt better, and received more services. One possible reason for this disparity in the research findings is that the populations screened were different. This would suggest that something more subtle and less costly is needed rather than blanket edicts from governments determining the frequency and content of screening for entire countries.

There is no evidence that routine blood-test screening of healthy people is effective in achieving any health objective—whatever the particular test (e.g. thyroxine, B_{12}, folate).

Perhaps the most important and constructive point to make here is to argue that our help for the elderly should be *targeted* to those in need.

Many other techniques have been explored with the aim of trying to find the most cost-effective way of detecting unreported problems. For UK readers working in British General Practice the government's recent legislation (1989) has made a comparison of these techniques of academic interest only, as the techniques to be employed have already been specified. For those readers working outside the UK we offer the following description of various screening techniques.

Method	Comment
1 GP carries out health check during ordinary consultations.	Puts great pressure on effective management of presenting problem; difficult to sustain.
2 GP carries out health check during clinic.	Time-consuming, inefficient, transport problems: not recommended.
3 Nurse carries out health check of individuals recruited during routine consultations.	More efficient than (2), but still problems with transport. Needs to be complemented by health checks of people who cannot come to the surgery. These can be done during domiciliary visits.
4 Completion of health-check form by elderly people, assisted by a voluntary helper.	Good system if you can recruit.
5 Elderly people complete a form in waiting-room, helped by a receptionist.	This allows problems to be identified but this can still be very time-consuming, unless the problems found can be referred to a 'clearing house', for example a liaison social worker or a volunteer.

Method	**Comment**
6 Elderly people sit at a VDU in the waiting room following on-screen prompts to give yes/no answers to life-style and social circumstances (e.g. the *Health Screen* for the Amstrad PCW).	Impossible for blind, confused, or demented people to manage the VDU—the very ones you want to identify. Helpful in giving the patient an overall summary of his health, which he can keep and refer to. May improve compliance and give rise to more truthful answers than face-to-face questioning (he cannot shock the computer).
7 Full assessment during a doctor-initiated home visit.	Very expensive in terms of time and manpower.

11 Organizational ideas from our own and other practices

How does the organization of a practice influence the quality of care it is able to give its elderly patients?

There are two main areas of organization: people and premises.

People

The practice nurse

The most useful job our practice nurse does in regard to the elderly is to run our weekly diabetic clinic (most of our diabetic patients are elderly). She is much better than we are at finding the time to teach patients about monitoring their own blood glucose. Ours is not the only practice to find that repetitive tasks which need meticulous attention such as filling in a diabetic co-operation card (ours is illustrated on p. 73 and shown again on the next page) are better performed by suitably trained nurses. We trained our own nurse in all items of diabetic care, including fundoscopy with a dilated pupil. We were rather uncertain about this latter activity—but teaching progressed satisfactorily until our efforts were overtaken by our ophthalmology department, which now screens patients regularly by retinal photography.

Here is a typical problem: the nurse is doing the clinic and finds that an elderly patient's blood pressure is 190/105 mmHg. She knows that it is practice policy for this sort of blood pressure not to be treated in the elderly—but what about in diabetic patients? She knows that blood-pressure control is important in diabetes. So she chooses a moment to put her head round my surgery door and ask for my opinion. I come out of my surgery and see the patient and come to a decision, e.g. that the patient should pay more attention to her diet, and by losing weight, control her blood pressure. The thought crosses my mind that it would have been easier to see the patient from the start myself—and this thought will be augmented if it transpires that the reason for poor dietary compliance is depression, and eating for solace following the death of her husband. This is one horn of a dilemma (*If you want a job done properly, do it yourself*). The other horn is *If a job can be delegated, delegate it*. These opposing views will find a slightly different resolution in each practice. In our practice we delegate a good deal, partly because we are lucky enough to have very good people working with us, and partly because, contrary to the negative thought expressed above, delegation *does* reduce the

Diabetic co-operation card

Name:	Address:	Telepone:		DOB	
Treatment:					
Date of diagnosis:		Is a consultant actively involved?			
Date seen by GP	/ /	/ /	/ /	/ /	/ /
Glucose, mmol/l:					
(WORST values)					
pre-breakfast	...	...	...	...	...
pre-lunch	...	...	...	...	...
pre-tea	...	...	...	...	...
pre-bed	...	...	...	...	...
other times	...	...	...	...	...
Weight (kg)	...	...	...	...	...
BP (mmHg)	...	...	...	...	...
Right-eye: acuity	...	...	...	...	...
cataract	...	...	...	...	...
dot/blots	...	...	...	...	...
new vessels	...	...	...	...	...
other	...	...	...	...	...
Left-eye: acuity	...	...	...	...	...
cataract	...	...	...	...	...
dot/blots	...	...	...	...	...
new vessels	...	...	...	...	...
other	...	...	...	...	...
Pupils dilated?	...	...	...	...	...
Dark room used?	...	...	...	...	...
Retinal photography	...	...	...	...	...
Urine [Protein]	...	...	...	...	...
Diet advice	...	...	...	...	...
Feet	...	...	...	...	...

work-load. It has to be said that if I had seen the elderly diabetic patient described above during the hurly-burly of ordinary surgery, I might not have remembered to take her blood pressure. If I did do her blood pressure, I could easily have been tempted to ignore my own rule and say to myself that no action was required. If I did have the time and energy to address the issue properly, who is to say that I would have elicited the fact that she was depressed, and that this was the reason for her over-eating? Our perception of a diabetic clinic is that it is somewhere where the care of diabetes goes on. But the patient's perception is often that the atmosphere is less rushed than normal surgery, and there is an opportunity to disclose more confidential matters.

Other practices delegate even more than we do. In the example given above the practice nurse may take it upon herself to refer the patient to a community psychiatric nurse, or she may undertake psychotherapy herself. Most of us think that this is the limit of delegation. Doctors are still needed, after all, for prescribing—which is often thought of as an insurmountable obstacle to further delegation. However, we know that in some dispensing practices the practice nurse *does* prescribe (according to routines agreed with the doctors). For this to work to the full, the practice needs to be a dispensing one. What happens is that the nurse writes the prescription, the dispenser dispenses it—leaving the prescription for the doctor to sign after surgery. The doctor may establish more control of prescribing by implementing the policy that certain groups of drugs can be prescribed this way, but cannot leave the dispensary without him checking the prescription. Alternatively, the nurse can discuss all her prescriptions at the end of surgery.

Even in non-dispensing practices, the practice nurse can do some prescribing—by writing prescriptions, giving them to the doctor to sign, and then taking them to the chemist the practice's patients usually use. In this way treatment is under way in 24–48 h—which is quite satisfactory for the treatment of chronic conditions, which are mostly what the nurse will be prescribing for (e.g. changing the dose of an oral hypoglycaemic agent in fine-tuning diabetic control).

The next most useful thing our practice nurse does for the elderly is to immunize many of them against influenza. Our initial practice was for her to be responsible (via the receptionist) for booking patients into her surgery—after instituting an 'advertising' campaign at the reception desk, and in the practice profile. This produced a gratifying but overwhelming response—there being so many elderly, well-informed patients in our practice that in October our nurse could do practically nothing else but immunize patients. So now our practice nurse's policy is to ask the receptionist to explain to patients when they phone in for 'flu immunization that there is heavy demand, and 'would you mind not having a personal appointment with the nurse, but to have the injection in a mass session in the waiting-room?—just come and roll up your sleeve. Everyone is coming at 2 o'clock. Do say if you would like an individual appointment.' It is clearly most important to make sure that the waiting-room is not going to be used for other purposes at the same time. So far, no patient has requested an individual appointment, and they seem to enjoy the organized chaos of a mass vaccination session. One patient commented with genuine nostalgia: 'It's like being back in the army—it's a great idea.' This, however, has served to warn us against too much regimentation. Normally our nurse will see 5–10 people per surgery—but on this scheme she can vaccinate 50 patients in half the time of the normal surgery. Originally it was thought that having the doctor vaccinating as well as the nurse would be the most efficient method—but we found we got in the way of the streamlined system developed by the nurse and the receptionist.

So now we have retired behind the desk in reception, to get on with paper work, while keeping a weather eye on the proceedings. Before the session begins, the receptionist gets out the patients' notes and puts them in alphabetical order, with a prescription ready written. She then replaces the waiting-room flowers with sharps bins. As the patients start arriving, she writes *Fluvirin* or *Influvac* (or whatever) in the notes, handing the patient their prescription and asking them to sign the back so that no prescription charge is payable. If a prescription charge is payable (our younger patients), she collects the money. (This is not necessary if the GP purchases the vaccinations—for which he or she is later reimbursed.) The patient then sits to be injected, and then hands the prescription to the nurse. We try and remember to tell everyone that we cannot guarantee that the immunization will be successful. The availability of single-dose injection units with the needle attached and vaccine drawn up ready is an important factor in speeding up our operations.

This system works adequately for those patients who are well-informed, motivated, and mobile. What about the house-bound and those who take less interest in their health, but who would benefit from influenza immunization? This is where a computer comes in useful in identifying at-risk patients.

Other practices flag the notes throughout the year of those patients attending for other matters who would benefit from influenza immunization, and then make sure that, by one method or another, they have all been immunized by the end of the autumn.

The Government's new scheme for visiting the elderly each year will create further opportunities for immunizations.

Our chemist supplies us in bulk with the 'flu injections *before* the prescription is signed (a financial liability for him and a great benefit to us). Other practices purchase their own injections, and make a small dose of large profits depending on any special deals made with distributors. This may be enough to finance the practice nurse's immunization sessions—but it only takes some adverse publicity, local (one of our patients died within hours of immunization) or national ('doctors have got the wrong strain of 'flu vaccine this year') for the purchasing GP to be left stranded with large numbers of 'flu injections which he has paid for, which no one wants, and for which he cannot be reimbursed.

The district (community) nurse

All practices will be familiar with the district nurse's most valuable contribution to the care of the elderly patients—the providing of 'all care' for the frail and dying in their own homes. But have there been any new and valuable initiatives extending her role? The most important such initiative is the provision, in some areas, of 24-hour, round-the-clock care. This greatly extends what the district nurse can do. The Peterborough experiment with the 'hospital-at-home' initiative extended this role even more—but this pattern has not been repeated in other areas of the UK, largely for logistic reasons. For example, there are disputes about who should foot the bill for prescribing, and about how medical (GP) cover should be arranged.

The health visitor

In all the practices we know, health visiting for the elderly is a custom more honoured in the breach than in the observance. Our own health authority does not have the energy to ensure the proper provision of Health Visitors. Because of cut-backs, underfunding, and unfilled but under-advertised posts our Health Visitor spends only two hours a week with the practice, making a mockery of the health-visiting ideal of service throughout the human life-cycle.

But what *could* the Health Visitor do for our elderly patients?

- Bereavement visiting
- Retirement counselling
- Screening for unrecognized or unmet health needs (p. 172)
- Encouraging fitness (p. 195)
- Setting up lunch clubs (a geriatric equivalent of mothers and toddlers groups).

The receptionists

The chief thing which elderly patients tell us that they value in their receptionist is a face and a voice which they recognize. Being welcomed by name by a familiar receptionist as soon as one enters the surgery is worth any amount of computer-generated patient details supplied by a faceless person operating behind a glass screen. And when a patient rings up in a panic, just hearing the voice of 'their' receptionist, whom they have known for many years and across many crises, has a more immediate and powerful tranquilizing effect than any amount of formal psychotherapy.

A skilled receptionist can help many of the logistic difficulties which elderly people face in getting health care.

- Taking prescriptions to the patient's nearest chemist.
- Explaining where to apply for benefits.
- Signing the back of prescriptions on behalf of elderly people to exempt them from prescription charges—if the patient is confused, and there is no other helper.
- During busy surgeries she can usher the elderly patient who is very slow and garrulous into a separate surgery, and help them undress (if required)—this is a real problem in the winter, with all the multitudes of coats, vests, and corsets. She can also aid the patient up on to the couch,

and adjust his hearing aid (if worn) so that time is used most effectively during the consultation. The doctor can indicate before or during surgery which patients are likely to need this help. But there is a danger which needs to be recognised when this streamlining of care is used: the doctor tends to take the history with the patient on the couch. This has two consequences. First, the doctor is then literally talking down to the patient—rather than on a one-to-one level. This may intimidate some patients, and the quality of the history may be impaired. The second factor is that, to the patient, it seems obvious that the examination is the key part of the consultaton, and he or she may forget to tell the doctor about important symptoms—particularly psychological symptoms. To get round these twin problems and yet retain the useful time-saving feature of this help from receptionists we favour the system whereby the doctor explains carefully what is going to happen to the patient. He may even choose to do the consultation in two stages—getting the patient back for a full examination. Another useful feature of this system is that when the patient is fully prepared by the receptionist, it does not take long to do an examination of the major bodily systems—and patients are often very grateful and reassured by this. If the receptionist stays in the room during the examination (with the patient's consent), the doctor can slip away after explaining the findings, leaving all the dressings, prolonged 'good-byes', and 'while I'm heres' for the receptionist to field. We may, of course, be missing vital information by not attending to 'while I'm here, doctor'—but the other side of the coin is that the patient now has an ally and confidante in the receptionist, and will not feel bad about asking 'What did the doctor mean by . . .?' Enquiries reveal that patients do not mind receptionists adopting this role, and it is a useful way for patients to build up trust with a central person in the primary care team.

- The receptionist can peform certain clinical tasks—such as doing ECGs. We recently bought an ECG without thinking that its automatic mode of operating was very important—it just seemed to add 'frill', and only just worth paying extra for. But we soon realized that this feature (whereby once the leads are in place, the whole operation is controlled by the push of one button once) meant that the receptionists could do ECGs. It is a simple matter to teach a receptionist where to put the leads—and just in case there is any mistake, we ask the receptionist to leave the leads on for us to check, while we are reading the ECG. Patients and receptionists seem to enjoy this extended role, and they may also enjoy the relaxed conversation with the receptionist while the procedure is being carried out. What to the doctor is an irritatingly time-consuming and rather messy exercise, is the highlight of some receptionist's day. They feel they are, and indeed they *are* contributing directly to patient-care. Nurses often have the role of doing ECGs, but may not be in the building when an ECG is needed (they often need doing at inconvenient times)—and if they are in the building, will have their own patients booked in, and it may not be satisfactory to squeeze in an 'emergency' extra. However, we still arrange for our nurse to do most of our 'elective' ECGs.

- Receptionists can also do dressings and ordinary first-aid procedures to at least as high a standard as most mothers (who would do these tasks without thought of involving a doctor). So it is a good idea to send one's staff on regular first-aid courses.

The pharmacist

The pharmacist is part of the primary health care team in its most extended form. He usually works from our own premises, and may not regard himself as part of any team. But from the patients' point of view he is another very frequently used professional who is easily accessible to turn to for advice. Here are some examples of how pharmacists and their assistants have helped our elderly patients in non-routine ways.

- By delivering drugs to the patient's home. This is the most useful service, and is a vital ingredient in looking after totally dependent patients, who are living alone in their own homes.
- 'Mr S has been in frequently to buy *Syndol*® (the over-the-counter pain-reliever which contains the highest dose of codeine phosphate). I thought he might be getting addicted, so when he was last in I refused to sell him any more, and suggested he came to see you.'
- 'I see that Mr X is on anti-TB treatment—do you think he should be taking pyridoxine to prevent isoniazid-induced neuropathy?'
- Agreement-forging between GP partners over the length of antibiotic courses. Once it is agreed how many days amoxycillin (for example) needs to be given for pneumonia, the pharmacist can make up bottles of tablets ready to be dispensed—so reducing waiting-times, and the need for the elderly patient to make two trips to the pharmacy (one to hand in the prescription, the other to pick up the drugs).

Patient's participation groups

The purpose of these is to harmonize the 'consumer's' and the 'provider's' aims through information and feedback about health and organizational matters. If a practice sets up a programme for the benefit of patients (e.g. mammography), it is very helpful to have feedback from the patients about its success, and ways of making the programme more acceptable. Patient participation groups are supposed to make known health needs of local people. In our practice, this rarely happens, and patients generally suppose that the general practitioner *is* the local person who knows the needs of patients. Complaints may also be aired in Patient Participation Group meetings, along with suggestions for improvements. The didactic role of the doctor in participation groups is hard to keep in perspective. Patients appear to like to have a lecture from their doctor on health matters. While this may be a good way of imparting information, it is hard to do in the spirit of participation—the central tenet of which is that the patient contributes to his or her own health care. Behind this central tenet is the assumption (which needs examining) that it is *healthier* if patients participate in their care, and that it is somehow wrong for everything to be handed to the patient on a plate. There is supposed to be some virtue in the process of striving for the best in health care. If it is worked for, it will be valued, and if it is valued it will be something that motivates the patient towards the more general proposition that he can influence his own destiny, and this in turn may augment a feeling of dignity and promote the optimism for the constructive activities on which positive health is based. In practice, however, few groups would be bold enough to say that they achieve or even aim for all these things. Our own group is moving towards this area by providing funds to buy equipment, and by lobbying politicians over inadequate or threatened services. Interestingly, both politicians and doctors claim to be the patient's advocate—so when they clash it is quite useful to be able to call on the only infallible authority on the goodness or otherwise of medical care: the patient himself (infallible, that is, so long as he is well informed).

Voluntary organizations

These extend in a practical way the benefits of participation outlined above. Each practice will exist within a unique framework of voluntary workers, so it is hard to make useful generalizations. Examples of useful voluntary help include a service of sitters to be with the dying and other solitary invalids; transport to day centres; domiciliary library services for the househound; and the running of lunch clubs for the bereaved or the single elderly.

Agencies such as the Guild for the Elderly and Age Concern frequently run local services. The local library is often a source of information about these and other services (such as which shops in the neighbourhood deliver to the home).

Repeat prescribing

This is one of the 'shop windows' of general practice in that it is a frequent source of contact with patients, and very much informs their judgement as to the approachability and standards of their general practice. With the elderly, it is a very common occurrence for the practice to be telephoned by the patient who starts a conversation which goes something like this: 'I'd like some more of my pills.' 'Which ones would you like?' 'What do you mean?

Just give me my usual tablets please.' The receptionist gets out the notes and finds that the patient is taking at least two drugs regularly, e.g. a diuretic and digoxin, and also pain killers for arthritis—so she asks the patient what they are for: 'Your heart or your arthritis?' 'You know, for my legs . . .' the patient replies. The receptionist interprets this is as a request for the arthritis tablets, whereas the patient's call to the surgery was prompted by swelling of her legs, and she thought she was asking for her diuretic. So the 'wrong' tablet is prescribed in spite of adequate records. This sequence demonstrates the truth of the maxim: *Everything tends to randomness*. How can this sort of problem be avoided? The purist will answer that this whole sequence shows that repeat prescribing should be abandoned. How does the realist respond? First, by saying that face-to-face contact is no insurance against randomness. We are all capable of misinterpreting what the patient wants. We might, for example, see the swollen legs and increase the dose of diuretic, without realizing that the patient had not been taking her diuretic *at all*. The result might be temporary improvement, followed by a worse state due to over-diuresis. The realist also responds by saying that if we abandoned all our repeat prescribing our surgeries would fill up, and become so busy that new mistakes would start to be made, and that existing aims would no longer be met. His strongest point, however would be to come up with a system that made such systems less likely. Computers are an aid in this regard, because they can automatically indicate when a particular prescription was last asked for. So, to return to our earlier example, the receptionist can call up the patient's details *while they are still on the telephone*. It takes only seconds to find which drugs are being prescribed on a regular basis, and which are 'one off' prescriptions. She can call up the patient's problem list equally quickly. It might read:

Osteoarthritis of hips . . . Responds to BD co-dydramol
Cardiac failure . . . Needs bendrofluazide regularly.

This enables the receptionist to ask the crucial question: 'Is it for your hips?' and 'When and how often do you take it?'. In other words, she has more information at her fingertips, so that she (or the doctor, if she passes the call to him) can ask the most accurate and discriminating questions. This system is theoretically possible with manual records. However, it often takes longer to go and find the records and turn up the relevant summaries. The lengthy task of data entry is the huge drawback to both systems, but the dividends are great: the doctor and the receptionist are more in control, and, if the computer system is used, audit is simplified. The practice manager, at the push of a few buttons, can create a group of all the patients with cardiac failure and then make sure that everyone has been requesting and receiving appropriate drugs.

Premises and locations

This is another important 'shop window' for general practice. If the surgery is central, and can afford easy parking, and if there are no steps, and plenty of ramps, very many old patients will find their way to surgery who would normally be regarded as 'house-bound'. If there is a non-appointments system, this helps too, as patients can choose to come when the weather is favourable, or if a friend or relative visits with a car a spontaneous outing to the doctor becomes possible.

We would all like to have pleasant, spacious, well-designed, fully equipped surgeries full of attractive and competent staff. But for many practices, particularly inner-city practices, this may seem an idle dream. Even such a basic task as keeping the premises clean may give rise to almost insuperable difficulties, if the surgery is in a decaying building, owned by a landlord who is not interested in improving his property. Vandalism and burglaries can, at a stroke, destroy months of painstaking work, leaving the practice demoralized and asking itself 'Why bother?' What advice is possible here? Grants and deprived-area allowances may be one solution—but this may not combat the demoralization that exists. What is needed is for the doctor to have protected time to plan and develop his services. If these activities are left till the end of the day, a busy evening surgery will subvert the best intentions and scupper any attempts at rational thought. One idea to combat this is for Family Health Services Authorities (FHSAs) to identify those practices in need, and offer to pay a locum for 5 hours a day for 6 months or whatever is required, so that the principal has protected time to analyse and develop his activities.

Finding the right premises is a key step to developing services. Buying and developing a site requires a huge investment of time (as well as money), and it is not surprising that not much gets done if these activities are squeezed in between impossibly busy surgeries. Once protected time is available, it may be possible to race through the following sequence:

- Ask the FHSA to declare your premises to be unsatisfactory.
- Identify a site.
- Approach the owner.
- Persuade him to consider a financial offer.
- Approach the FHSA to give an informal opinion as to the site's feasibility.
- Get a loan from a finance house.
- Get planning permission for change of usage.
- Draw up contracts for the purchase of the site.
- Exchange contracts.
- Engage an architect.
- Refine and re-plan as needed.
- Show plans to the FHSA.
- Get plans approved by the district medical officer.

- Find at least three builders.
- Get competitive tenders.
- Start building or converting
- Arrange supervision of stage payments to the builder (so that if he goes out of business you have not paid for more than you have got).
- Have the new building approved by architects and FHSA.
- Arrange for every patient to be told in writing of your proposed move.
- Move into new or converted buildings.

If the above sequence is adhered to, the purchase of the site may be arranged (in the UK) under the 'cost rent scheme'. Under this scheme the practice owns the building and the FHSA pays the practice a rent which is not a commercial rent—but a rent set at a higher level to take account of all the development costs (but not the capital cost of the land)

What has all this got to do with the care of the elderly? This question is like asking what adult literacy has got to do with maternal mortality. Someone who is very keen to reduce maternal mortality might try the direct approach: employing more doctors and midwives, or giving extra training to anaesthetists. We know that this does not have much effect on maternal mortality in the Third World. A 2 per cent increase in direct resources yields very little return. But a 2 per cent increase in adult literacy has a very marked effect on maternal mortality. The motto is: *Do not make your care-initiatives too focused*. Local circumstances may make initiatives directed specifically at the elderly of very limited value, when what is needed is to break out of a mould which influences whole areas of your practice—and then the standard of care goes up for everyone, and so, incidentally for the elderly.

How to use a cyclical five-year plan

We have been in the position of over-pressed general practitioners from an underdeveloped practice looking with envy and some distaste (born out of having to make a virtue out of necessity) at the smooth operations of a well-capitalized practice with plenty of partners, attached staff, equipment, and ideas. We know the feeling of hopelessness on returning to our own practice, where everything tends towards randomness. Where do you start—when it is so uphill in every direction? It may be helpful to indicate that the start can be made *at any point* in the cycle illustrated below. It is also necessary to indicate that there is no need to try and do everything at once. This may lead to repeated failures and further demoralization. It probably takes five years to go round the cycle illustrated below. Then give yourself five years off (call it time for assessment and consolidation)—and then go round the cycle again, starting anywhere and finishing up with more assessment and consolidation.

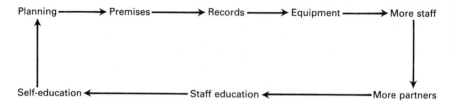

Side-effects

Once upon a time our practice consisted of a single-handed doctor, a receptionist, and a district nurse all working out of a rented shop. Now we have more than doubled the number of partners and district nurses. In addition we have a practice nurse, more receptionists, a computer operator, and a secretary—all working out of purpose-built premises. These we have gained. But what have we lost? Does the fairy story have a happy ending? Twentieth-century pharmacology has taught us one important thing: whatever the intervention, there are *always* side-effects to be felt somewhere in the system.

What are the side-effects of changing a simple, homespun activity into an industry? Loss of the personal approach; loss of continuity; a dilution of responsibility and an ending of a single coherent source of advice for patients. These problems will be felt all the more keenly by the vulnerable members of the practice list: the old, the inadequate, and the disadvantaged—but they may be mitigated by such devices as personal lists, job descriptions with demarcated responsibilities, agreed practice policies on common problems, and a willingness to get to know patients personally.

One of the key aims is to foster a happy atmosphere in the practice so that everyone enjoys the work, and staff are not continually leaving to take up new appointments.

12 How can your local geriatric hospital help?

In order to run an effective service for the elderly in general practice it is an enormous help to have a Geriatric Department which is flexible and able to respond quickly to the needs of one's patients. It might be thought that the general practitioner is either blessed with a good department or a bad department—and that there is not much he or she can do to influence things either way. But this is not the case—as this chapter will demonstrate. The running of a good geriatric department is very much a partnership between consultant geriatrician and general practitioner. The two most telling tests of any geriatric department are: *can this ill elderly patient be admitted today?*—and, when the time for discharge comes: *will the discharge fail, and the patient be re-admitted, or abandoned?*

How can a geriatric hospital gear itself up to provide more available beds, especially when resources are falling? We here produce a blueprint which enables bed availability to be increased by an order of magnitude—with admissions sometimes exceeding 25 patients per 65 000 elderly per day (rather than per month—which was formerly the case). The rate at which this transformation can be achieved is detailed in Table 12.1 and Fig. 12.1. During the period illustrated in the graph the total number of beds available *fell* by 24 per cent in the Health Authority concerned (Worthing). In spite of this there were 4189 admissions in 1987 compared with just 352 admissions in 1974. The local geriatricians and general practitioners can work together on the following areas to enable this to happen.

The move away from custodial care

Custodial care in its pure form is now not practised by any geriatric department. On this model, the geriatrician fills his beds with patients who do not want to or cannot go home. When a request comes in for an acute admission for someone who has had a stroke (for example) he says 'My beds are all occupied—but I will put Mrs Smith down on the waiting-list.' The waiting-list may be in double or even triple figures, and the geriatrician cannot say when a bed will be available *because death is the only way of releasing a bed.*

If, over the next few months, an influenza epidemic stalks the geriatric wards beds become available at a rate which enables Mrs Smith to climb to the top of the waiting list. The great day arrives for her to be admitted to

Table 12.1 Geriatric yearly statistics

	Admissions	Discharges and deaths
1974	352	278
1975	502	450
1976	696	674
1977	1126	1071
1978	1459	1440
1979	1810	1687
1980	2213	2238
1981	2700	2606
1982	3101	3029
1983	3705	3661
1984	3682	3768
1985	3748	3578
1986	3958	3822
1987	4189	4150
1988	4178	4170
1989	4275	4210

hospital. But by this time, spasticity and contractures have set in, and no amount of physiotherapy will make her independent. Mrs Smith, who was once only in need of a week or two of intensive rehabilitation, is now a long-stay custodial case.

The Lingam–Aal formula

The way out of the above impasse is to have direct access to beds for GPs, and to abolish the waiting-list. Then Mrs Smith can get the rehabilitation she needs when she needs it. The nurses can see that their efforts are rewarded. Doctors know that their diagnoses are important and they realize that the fine-tuning of their clinical skills *does* produce results. (Some Mrs Smiths turn out to have subdural haemorrhages, the alert clinician will discover.) The medical work is seen as challenging—so a better quality of junior staff is attracted. This leads to more cures—so more discharges and more beds, more admissions, more clinical experience, and still more cures. This sounds just like the sort of positive cycle that does not occur in practice, and nobody well-versed in the degradation of clinical ideals when confronted by the real world would be bold enough to put forward such a positive cycle to a unit manager as an argument for more fully-trained nurses. So it is very surprising

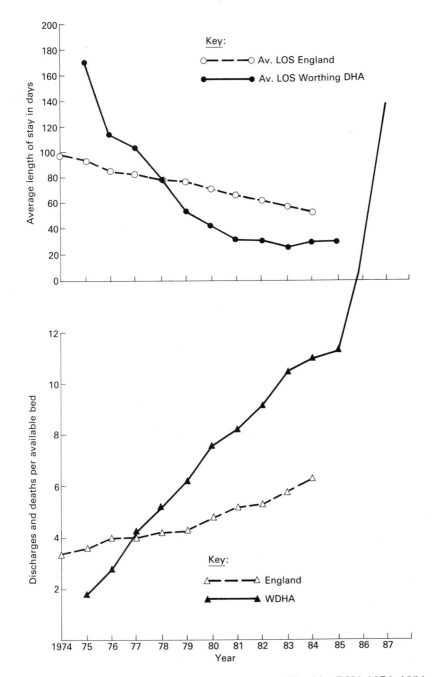

Fig. 12.1 Changes in geriatric bed usage, England and Worthing DHA 1974–1984.
Sources: SH3 Annual returns DHSS Statistical Bulletin 5/85

to learn that in the real world such a positive cycle *can* occur, as illustrated in Fig. 12.1.

It is hard to interpret Fig. 12.1 unless the death-rate is known and the readmission-rate is known. A sceptic might say that nothing has been achieved if the 4189 admissions for 1987 consisted in 350 patients (the admission figure for 1974), each admitted and readmitted over ten times during the course of the year. One reply to the sceptic would be to point out that even if the readmission-rate is high, this does not negate the whole exercise—as the patient is at least able to spend half his time at home. A better answer is to quantify the readmission-rate exactly, and let the figures speak for themselves. For the figures given in the accompanying tables, the death-rate is 25 per cent and the readmission rate is 11 per cent—the latter being less than that for most general hospital admissions.

Abolishing the waiting-list

How is this possible? If one looks at the reasons why long-stay patients are not going home, a very common reason is that relatives have had such a struggle before the patient was finally admitted to hospital that they are most reluctant to countenance the return of the patient. Although they may be able to cope with the patient when she is relatively well, as soon as any problem occurs, they fear that they will not be able to cope—and that there will be no one to take the relative off their hands should the need arise.

The way forward is to promise the relatives that if things go wrong, a bed will be available *within 24 hours*. This might seem to be a very courageous or even foolish thing to do. You may find yourself with an army of aggrieved relatives and a full hospital. All that can be said is that since the geriatricians at Worthing Hospital started making this promise ten years ago, bed availability has gone up dramatically—*and the promise has never been broken*.

Direct access to beds

For some GPs this will seem like an impossible dream—just to pick up the telephone and ask a secretary to arrange to admit your patient within 8 hours. No questions are asked (apart from formalities) and there is no questioning of one's clinical judgement. Surely such a system is open to great abuse. The lazy GP would be on the telephone all the time—and have a very easy life. In Worthing this does not seem to have materialized. What *has* happened is that geriatric patients can be admitted from day 1 of the illness, when the prospect of cure is at its highest.

An important psychological shift has also occurred. If the general practitioner knows that he can get his patient admitted in 8 hours if necessary, he will be more prepared to try treatment at home if this is what the patient would prefer. He can afford to risk things going wrong if he or she has prompt back-up.

Setting up a system of direct access to beds by GPs requires some investment in secretarial time. A geriatric office needs to come into being, with the telephone manned promptly throughout the working day. With three or four hospitals on different sites which can admit patients, the geriatric office has to be fed with fast facts about bed-occupancy two or three times a day.

During the emergence of open access to GPs, an important precept appeared: the GP should ask for what he wants. If the patient needs admission, we should ask for an admission—not a domiciliary visit by a geriatrician. This leaves the geriatrician free to spend time on the wards and in the homes of those who decline hospital admission, or who are not admitted for other reasons.

How much of the excess throughput that the implementation of these ideas achieves is dependent on discharging patients to nursing homes and Part III accommodation? About 60 per cent of discharges are to home (i.e. the place where the patient came from). This means that it *is* useful—but not essential—to have a range of options for discharge from hospital—to rest homes, local authority homes, warden-controlled flats, and nursing homes.

13 Helping older people to live at home

One of the main objectives of those providing care for older people is to help those older people who want to, to live at home—and to do so with as much dignity as possible.

The purpose of this chapter is to describe the contribution general practitioners can make to best achieve this objective. The roles of the district nurse and the occupational therapist are described elsewhere (p. 180) and pp. 209–15).

Let us start with a patient:

Miss M. was disabled with arthritis and had in addition a 'difficult' personality made apparently worse by intermittent deafness, which had all combined to rather alienate neighbours and professional helpers. One day she was admitted to hospital with pneumonia, and remained in hospital for a long time. When the time came for discharge it was discovered that both her heating and her cooking appliances were defective, and she was therefore discharged without adequate heating or cooking facilities. Attempts to solve these problems became confused, with each agency suggesting that the other had failed to help Miss M. After several cold nights at home feeling unsupported and vulnerable she finally 'agreed' to go into residential care. The energy required for fighting to achieve a comfortable and safe environment was too great for her.

Miss M. illustrates at least nine of the major problems which beset old people who are trying to live an independent life at home.

1 Loss of the ability to look after oneself and perform the activities of daily life; this leads to either deprivation or dependence on others.
2 Insufficient income.
3 Housing in poor repair, or in need of improvement, or difficult to heat adequately.
4 Involvement of a multiplicity of agencies and professionals.
5 Social isolation.
6 Sensory deprivation.
7 Health problems which affect the old person's ability to relate to other people, for example psychiatric illness, hearing and visual problems, dysphasia, and difficulties with mobility.
8 Chronic medical problems which impair the quality of life although they do not affect the old person's domestic abilities—for example, pain, depression, or incontinence.
9 A sense of suffering and hopelessness owing to such factors as:
   • The loss of humour (the causes of this are explored on p. 40).

- Dependence on others.
- The attitudes of those on whom the old person is dependent.
- For those who are religious, a sense of hurt or injustice that 'God has let this happen to me.'
- A sense of guilt due to the belief that the problem is a punishment for past sins.

Let us look at some of these points in more detail.

Loss of the ability to look after oneself

Check-list to help reverse disabilities

- Have I diagnosed all the diseases which are relevant?
- Do I know the exact cause of this old person's disability?
- Is the old person taking all necessary treatment?
- Is the dose sufficient? Or too much?
- Are there psychological factors impairing the patient's motivation.
- Could a physiotherapist help her regain the skill?
- Could an occupational therapist help the old person by adapting the house, her appliances, or her utensils, or by teaching new skills?

If the answer to all these questions is negative then it is appropriate to refer the old person for a service which does things for her. This may seem a counsel of perfection; but this type of review can be done relatively quickly, and can make a very important contribution to helping older people maintain health and well-being by helping them to keep *active*. Good evidence is now accumulating that exercise and fitness are of central importance—as revealed by the Fitness and Health Advisory Group of the Sports Council in studies in conjunction with the Health Education Authority (Gloag 1990). The first validation of exercise programmes from this new group (Professor Fentem's Activity and Health Research Group) are now being made available. They have found that a staggering 52 per cent of all those over 60 were *completely or virtually inactive*. Here is a cycle which leads to ever-increasing cardio-respiratory idling and social dependency.

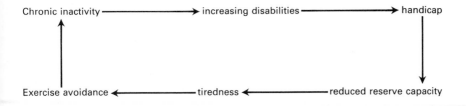

Insufficient income   No one can keep up with all the changes that take place in Social Security regulations. All that most of us have time to do is:

- To know the main benefits that are available to disabled people, notably the Attendance Allowance, and the Invalid Care Allowance—in UK practice.
- Be willing to encourage the older person to apply for such benefits, and to dispel any idea that they are 'charity'.
- If necessary, make contact so that someone can visit the old person to help them sort out their income problems.

Housing problems   Housing legislation is also extremely complex. There are only a small number of agencies to bear in mind when seeing an old person at home who has housing problems. Council tenants or housing association tenants can be helped by the landlord, who is obliged to maintain the property, repair it, improve it (sometimes), and may, on the advice of an occupational therapist, adapt it to minimize the impact of disability.

Private tenants and owner occupiers will find that the Environmental Health Department is the best source of help, because each Environmental Health Department has a housing section whose members are experienced in dealing both with elderly people and with the reluctant landlord.

Social isolation   Social isolation can cause or aggravate:

- Depression
- Anxiety
- Paranoia
- Confusion

Isolation may simply be a continuation of an isolated life-style—so the biography of the old person is important to take into consideration; but if it is a new feature in the life of an old person it is usually caused by disabling disease, for example sensory deprivation or immobility, or psychiatric disease, particularly Alzheimer's disease.

There are three steps which can be taken to minimize the impact of social isolation:

- Increasing the number of trips out of the home.
- Increasing the number of visitors to the home.
- Increasing stimulation within the home, for example by giving the old person a pet.

Social isolation is a difficult problem to tackle because there is no agency which counts this among its chief responsibilities. Referral of a socially isolated old person to social services will not usually result in effective action, except where the local authority has day-centre facilities. Sometimes, however, the very people who are most socially isolated are too disabled to be acceptable at the local authority day centre—and these same people are often excluded from day-hospital provision because they need long-term support.

The general practitioner should be aware of voluntary visiting and day-centre schemes organized either by local old people's clubs or the local branch of Age Concern, or some other similar voluntary organization. Depending on work-load and local circumstances, either the district nurse or the health visitor may be willing to help individuals who are socially isolated. This is so easy to write in a book, and so hard to accomplish in the field. For example, we have had reports of health visitors expressing enthusiasm for helping the elderly in their patch. They devise a questionnaire and a programme of visiting for those over 70 years old. The GP provides them with a full list, whereupon the truth sinks in that the numbers involved are far too great. The threshold is increased to 80 years old, and then to 85 years to make the numbers manageable. At this point a government directive comes to all health visitors to take on some new and pressing work with children (say, the prevention of cot-deaths)—and the whole project has to be shelved. This is an example of the best intentions evaporating under the intense heat generated when conflicting priorities grind against each other—with the inevitable result that old people miss out because they are worth less (p. 35).

One way to mitigate this might be to have one member of the primary health care team whose *only* responsibility is the social well-being of the elderly. There is some evidence that such a post might be too boring to attract those of suitable calibre; but we feel that the possibility is worth exploring. How civilized are we? What have we achieved with all our wealth, our computing, our technology, and our post-war philosophy? The answer lies in how we treat those who miss out because they are of low priority. Prioritizing is the rational activity of those who are under siege or who are about to sink ('Women and children first'). As conditions become more favourable, such a philosophy looks more and more grotesque. In these circumstances, an argument can be put forward for *inverting* lists of priorities. Here is a simple list of priorities which might have existed in an average practice in, say, 1985—in the fairly uncontroversial order given below:

1 Defibrillators for all treatment rooms (would save 500–600 lives a year).
2 Computers on every GP's desk (would provide invaluable audit material for enriching very many activities).
3 Sterile instruments for performing a wide range of small operations (this would cut down hospital waiting-times, and would be very popular with patients).
4 A practice nurse specifically for the elderly (this would fill a definite gap).

Simple planning philosophy says: 'Start at the top of the list; work downwards until the money runs out.' This is what practice A does. New money and new priorities arrive. Item number 3 is always towards the bottom of every list. It never quite materializes. Practice B, which is not happy with the siege mentality described above, *inverts* this list—on the very interesting assumption that *top-priority items contain their own energy*, and will generally achieve themselves, on account of being high-profile and vital. This practice takes the risky action of starting off by appointing a nurse for the elderly—with the partners saying to themselves 'items one and two are likely to come anyway: we do not know how exactly. So let us start with the last item on our list.'

How do practice A and B compare after 5 years? Practice A has a defibrillator and computer system which is capable of providing terminals on every desk. Some extra terminals have been bought, but 75 per cent of the way towards the goal of total computerization, the money ran out (so the trainee and the practice manager had to share terminals). So in 1990 there is no practice nurse for the elderly, an incomplete set of surgical instruments, and not a little frustration over VDUs.

Practice B has a nurse for the elderly. Its money ran out at this point (both practices have the same budget)—and it looked as though there were not going to be any defibrillators at least in 1985. But then the British Heart Foundation supplied one on loan, free of charge, as part of a national scheme, having decided that this was a highly cost-effective way of using its donated monies. As the year wore on, a company loaned them a full computer system with 6 VDUs on a 'no-cost' option ('no-cost' because the commercial company uses and sells the anonymized data generated by the computer to pharmaceutical firms and government departments). The next year practice B could afford a full set of surgical instruments. By 1989 practice B had realized its list of objectives in full. By 1990, practice B's health authority started supplying its general practitioners with sets of sterile instruments for a nominal charge which only reflected the cost of sterilization, and not the capital cost. Practice B was now able to sell practice A (which was in a different Health Authority) its complete set of surgical instruments. Practice B now has a small surplus and can afford to set a new set of priorities.

This saga illustrates more than the well-known point that in business, the winner takes all: it illustrates that priorities *do* have energies. The right lesson to learn is too simply expressed as 'start at the bottom and work up'—because the practice might have put something absurd as the last item on the list. The more sophisticated approach is to make a list of priorities, and then score them on a seven-point scale of desirability—and then to score them on a similar score according to their perceived internal energy, with 7 representing the most inertia, and 1 representing the least inertia. If this looks like a conjuring trick to give extra priority to those of us with special axes to grind in the field of geriatrics, we should respond by saying that we would be quite happy to be 'out-prioritized' by items with even more inertia than geriatric medicine—for example, the homeless or those with intractable mental illness.

Table 13.1 Priority-scoring with compensation for inertia

	Desirability	Inertia*	Total score
1 Defibrillators	7	0	7
2 Computers	5	3	8
3 Instruments	4	2	6
4 Nurses for the elderly	3	7	10

* As defined above.

It should not be thought that the central tenet of this form of prioritizing *depends* on items with high internal energies somehow arriving free on the GP's desk. In the above examples the free energy did indeed manifest itself in this way, but this energy could equally well have manifested itself as energy to motivate the GP to buy equipment, find the time for a special activity, or to hire staff to increase services. Here is an entirely different example from a different sphere of general practice. Seeing the sick who present themselves to surgery is, very understandably, our top priority. Dr C. is on his way to morning surgery when it occurs to him that a short detour will lead him to the home of Mrs Y. whose elderly mother had died in hospital twenty-four hours earlier. On a simple reading of his priorities he should drive on and see his sick patients, who he knows will already be queuing for his services. If there is any time over at the end of the day, non-essential tasks such as unsolicited visits may be slotted in. However, Dr C. knows that there is really no such thing as 'the end of the day': he will go on working until the last sick patient has been seen, and once the last patient has been seen his top priority (quite rightly) is to free himself from the day's vicissitudes by rest and recreation. In this example of Dr C. driving to morning surgery, seeing the bereaved daughter is the low-priority option, but one which is also of very low internal energy, and attending to the sick is an option of high priority, but also one of such high internal energy that it can be delayed without risk of default. If Dr C. is under siege (a concurrent influenza epidemic) he may choose to pass by Mrs Y. and let her take a chance with all the other items of secondary importance that are likely never to get done. In other circumstances, and if he uses our method of inverting priorities, Mrs Y. is more likely to get a visit (if she is in).

Various objections may be levelled at the system of thinking which leads to the inverting of lists of priorities. For example, what would happen if *every-one* used this system—including the British Heart Foundation in the earlier example above? If this charity gave providing defibrillators an overall priority which was lower than some other of its aims, on the grounds that this priority had sufficient internal momentum to realize itself without their help? Useful points to make in countering this argument are that, in the first place, it is extremely unlikely that everyone would use the system of thought outlined above. Secondly, even if the British Heart Foundation had used this system of prioritizing, it is quite likely that some other charity or body would have filled the gap—or have been brought into existence *solely* to fill this gap.

Sensory deprivation   The problems of visual and hearing impairment are described on p. 132 and p. 82 respectively. The effect of these impairments on elderly cognitive processes is further described on p. 38.

Suffering and hopelessness   Older patients often have multiple problems which interrelate in complex and confusing ways. It is important, however, not to overlook the fact that the old person with greatest need may simply need to relate to someone they trust, someone with whom they can discuss their feelings of uselessness and redundancy, or their feelings of unfairness that a particular disability should have happened to them, or that death has removed their spouse—when so many around them appear healthy and well. For many elderly people, their experience of disease is not only a source of physical problems such as those expressed in the question 'Why me?' Unfortunately, health and social services and the professionals who work within them are trained to deal with discrete physical problems, and may be embarrassed when older people raise more profound issues. There is a part to play for churches and priests or holy men of any religion or denomination, and in many cases the gap between the primary care team and local religious organizations is too wide. Elderly people fall through this gap, being referred to the priest too late for anything but the last rites.

Useful opening questions for older patients are:

'You have such a lot of problems, I do not know if you ever wonder why this has all happened to you, or if you just accept it all as bad luck?'

'What do you make of all these problems that you have got? Some older people are very puzzled by the fact that these problems have happened to them, particularly if they are religious; I don't know if this ever bothers you?'

Whatever the doctor believes himself, it is important to offer these openings to older people, and to give them the opportunity of raising broader issues about suffering—which may be equally, if not more, important to them than the details of their drug regime or the details of their income and how it can be increased.

Problem-solving

Although each problem has to be tackled in a different way, there are some principles of problem-solving which may be useful, particularly in helping trainees come to terms with the complex problems they encounter when working with older people. Their problem-solving may be considered to be a cycle as shown in the diagram below.

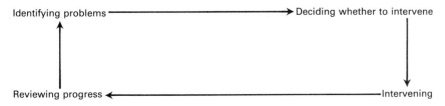

Identifying problems   Some problems are easily identified. The old person seeks a consultation with the problem that is bothering them most, and describes it clearly to the general practitioner. However, not all problems come easily packaged, and two aspects of health in old age have to be taken into account when planning a problem-based approach for general practice. One is how to elicit unreported problems from people who rarely visit their doctor. The other factor to take into account is that simply taking a full history may not be enough. It is often vitally important to question a relative or neighbour. A number of features should be an integral part of consultations with old people.

- Fully informing older people about the possibilities for action.
- Discussing whether something really is a problem or not.
- Checking through a list of self-care and mobility problems to complete a comprehensive assessment of disability.
- Asking the opinion of other people—and then (sometimes) reflecting this back to the patient as an aid to increasing sight.

Guidance for trainers

Problem solving is one aspect of work with older people that trainees may need help with. If he or she is likely to have worked in a Geriatric Medical Unit, they will have received some training in this approach. However, it cannot be assumed that communication skills have been assessed, and, if necessary, improved. On the contrary, there is good evidence that communication skills are actually lost during medical training. Helpful techniques for trainers to consider are:

- Interviewing the old person after the trainee has done so, but in ignorance of the findings.

- Analysis of a video recording of a consultation.
- The development of a check-list of the activities mentioned above for the trainee to use in advance, to plan consultations.
- Giving the trainee the opportunity to discuss the problems identified or missed after a consultation.

Deciding whether or not to intervene   It is easy to identify problems in old age, but it is more difficult to help an older person to take a decision on whether or not intervention is worth while. It is important to remember that there is a distinction between decision-making—namely, weighing up pros and cons—and decision-taking, namely the final decision to act or not to act. In theory, the older person should always be the decision-taker, with the doctor simply helping with the making of the decision by comparing and enlarging the options available. But this theory does not work out very well in practice. Some older people with, say, Alzheimer's disease, are totally incompetent and are unable to weigh up evidence. There is a grey area between this state of affairs and a state of total lucidity (to which few of us aspire) and independence of thought in which the opinion of the doctor is of no special interest to the patient. It is in this grey area between these extremes that ethical problems abound—and which are discussed more fully in Chapter 11.

Considering the benefits, costs, and risks of intervening   The doctor should consider the following variables, and ask the following questions.
    Natural history: 'What is likely to happen to this person if we do not treat him or her?'

In the simplest type of condition, people affected deteriorate steadily until either they die or they start getting steadily better. More often a difficult decision arises because a proportion of people left untreated will not suffer any adverse effects. Not all heavy smokers get lung cancer—however long they have smoked. Only a few people with a symptomless abdominal aortic aneurysm will suffer a leak.

    The probability of benefit: 'What is the likelihood that this particular patient will benefit from this treatment?'
    The magnitude of the benefit. 'Even if this treatment works, how big will the actual benefit be to my patient?'

The magnitude of the benefit varies from treatment to treatment, and from patient to patient—in ways it is hard to predict.

    The probability of side-effects: 'What are the risks associated with this treatment?'

Balancing benefits and risks requires first of all some estimate of the probability that adverse side-effects will occur. Often this balancing act depends on comparing like with unlike (adding months of life with some pain, or a swifter death, say). In this sort of case decisions often have to be taken 'off the top of one's head'.

The magnitude of the side-effects: 'Just what will happen if things do not work out well?'

An uncommon side-effect which is fatal would normally be much more significant than a common trivial side-effect. But in some patients this may not be the case. There is an eighty-year old patient in our practice with intractable tinnitus—unrelenting, totally occupying, and continually torturous—which is made a little bit better by very large doses of amitriptyline—so large that the patient has a dry mouth and blurred vision, just to complete his hell. Such a person might leap at the offer of cochlear nerve transection, knowing full well that the result will be permanent deafness with the added possibility of a fatal outcome of the procedure. Death or deafness without tinnitus would, to him, be bliss.

The patient's point of view   Clearly, the aim should be to achieve some sort of harmony between the patient's and the doctor's point of view—and well-informed patients will ask questions like those we have portrayed the doctor asking him/herself in the preceding section. These questions, of course, relate to the main headings in the health-belief model, which states that people take into account:

- The seriousness of the condition.
- Their own susceptibility to developing it.
- The possibility that they will benefit if they follow their doctor's advice.
- The cost of following their doctor's advice, whether this is financial cost or inconvenience or the risk of adverse effects.

However, these decisions that an old person has to take is influenced not only by these factors, but also by their attitudes and expectations, and older people tend to have:

1 Lower material standards than younger people, because they have known much harder times; this may allow them to accept a situation which younger people would define as a problem that must be tackled at once.
2 Expectations which are not so high; many old people have known a large number of disappointments in their lifetime—and taking a decision to seek a solution for their problem requires an expectation that success is a possibility. Many elderly people have had so many disappointments, including disappointments from professionals, that they prefer to say 'I'm all right', rather than expose themselves to yet another disappointment.
3 A less well-defined view of their rights than young people, so that they are not so prepared to seek solutions to problems which require an individual to challenge authority.

Finally, old people may be reluctant to admit that they have a problem for fear that the recognition of a problem will lead to pressure to enter a home or institution being applied. It may be safer to say 'I'm all right', even if you are not, than admit you have a problem to someone who says they can help you, unless you are absolutely clear that what they mean by 'help' is not a place in a residential home, but the type of help you want in the place you want it.

Activities involved with decision-making   It is useful to help trainees think about the activities involved in decision-making and decision-taking, and to reflect upon their own level of competence in these particular activities.

- Informing the older person of the full range of options. This requires a good imagination, as well as good knowledge of the availability of local services—and those further away, which may be brought into the sphere of the old person's life. For example, if the patient wants a new hip in time to visit her Canadian grandchildren in the summer, you will need to know where the shortest waiting-list is this side of the Atlantic. The doctor also needs to have a good knowledge of his patient. One sort of patient may think that the doctor is rather mad to recommend yoga to help with their headaches—whereas for another person, this may be just what is needed.
- Informing the older person about the risks and benefits of different types of treatment.
- Listening.
- Allowing the older person time and the opportunity to discuss options with a third party.
- Involving a third party in discussion—for example, a trusted son or daughter.
- Giving clear advice on what the general practitioner thinks is the most appropriate courses of action—and *why*.

Helping trainees acquire these skills   Trainees can be helped to acquire these skills by:

- Preparing information on risks and benefits before a consultation.
- Recording the questions the old person asks during a consultation—for later discussion with the trainer.
- Laying aside time for reflection with the trainer and discussion with him or her of the way in which a decision was reached by an old person.
- Giving the trainee practice with common clinical problems by asking him or her to present options to the trainer. The type of clinical problem that can be used includes:

   The discovery of a symptomless aortic aneurysm of about 5 cm diameter in a man aged 74.

A report of gallstones in someone who has not been complaining of classic symptoms of gall-bladder disease.

Blood-pressure readings with a systolic consistently over 180 mmHg and a diastolic consistently over 105 mmHg in a woman aged 73 years.

Intervening

Having taken a decision that the benefits of intervention are likely to be greater than the risks and costs to the elderly person, the doctor has then to intervene to bring about change. This involves a number of activities, some of which are activities classically taught in medical schools; but there are other aspects which are likely to need as great an emphasis when dealing with older people. These include:

- Tailoring the prescribing to fit the unique predicament of the patient.
- Encouraging the old person to change their life-style or to try to overcome their disability.
- Giving advice to the old person about ways in which they could cope, and showing how objectives can be broken down into small attainable items of behaviour. This activity is sometimes called counselling.
- Trying to help older people reconcile fundamental differences with family or friends; for example, helping the old person tell her daughter that she wants to stay at home, even though she knows that she is at risk, or to help the daughter tell the elderly parent that she is too tired to visit her every day, and that she must accept home help and meals on wheels.
- Setting objectives.
- Recording baseline measurements against which change or lack of it can be measured.
- Arranging follow up as appropriate.

Helping trainees   When helping trainees develop their skills it is necessary not only to try to encourage trainees to take a fundamental approach to the problems of older people—for example, focusing on disabilities rather than diseases or biochemical criteria of 'normality'. It is also important to encourage a problem-solving approach. When working with older people the aim should be to try and identify all the problems that need to be tackled, and to set out objectives for each problem, and then to plan appropriate follow-up for each problem.

Recording objectives and planning follow up   A problem-based approach to clinical practice can be facilitated by giving some thought to the way in which information is collated and recorded. The conventional approach to record-keeping often makes it difficult to relate outcomes to a particular problem, because the follow-up consultation is recorded in the lines below those lines used to record problems. A problem–objective sheet can help focus attention on the most important problems, and facilitate a systematic approach to follow-up. The practice might consider developing their own sheets, such as the sheet shown below.

Health problem	Criteria used to measure severity	Present position	Target objective agreed with patient	Review date	Position on review	Action, e.g. close this problem, or carry forward to new sheet

Fig. 13.1 Objective-orientated medical record.

Objective-orientated medical records

We have spent some time trying to use this type of record in our practice—its attraction being that it is possible to see what the outcome of a particular problem has been. Clearly, such a record could only be used in selected patients—or else Monday morning's surgery would not have finished by Friday evening. The main problem with this system is that you can only fit one or two problems on a card—particularly if the criteria used to measure severity are multiple. Also, it is often hard to distinguish usefully between the criteria used to measure the severity, and the target. It is also a record that can only be used twice; the first time the patient presents (the column marked

'Present position;) and a second time ('Position on review'). This is wasteful in general practice, when patients may be seen hundreds of times for the same problem. These difficulties are magnified when it is appreciated that problems often undergo subtle changes in definition as time goes by—so that when the patient comes for review you find yourself trying to ram a square peg into a round hole.

We have found it useful to circumvent some of these problems by using computer software which enables one to tag any problem with a comment and a priority, from 0 to 9. At the push of two keys (H1), one can then review the patient's main problem (priority 1). Pushing keys H2 then gives one a different set of problems—and so on. This is quite useful in making the screen uncluttered, but the software does not allow one to review *only* say, priority 5 items: it will only give you priorities $\geqslant 5$. A problem with this approach is that if there is an almost insignificant addition to the chief problem, it has to be coded as priority one, when in fact the item concerned is of very low intrinsic priority. Perhaps the best solution would be to add a letter after each entry to denote which item on the problem list the entry referred to. Keying H1C would then reveal all the priority one items relating to problem C.

The problems underline the fact that there is no very satisfactory way of recording *all* consultations and interventions. We suspect that the main use for objective-orientated medical records will be as an idea in the mind of the doctor—rather than a reality in a Lloyd-George NHS envelope. The main value of this idea is that, with difficult patients, it will prompt us to ask ourselves: what is the objective, and how am I going to measure progress towards it?

Reviewing progress

Follow-up action to review the impact of intervention completes the first treatment cycle. It involves the following activities:

- Arranging a follow-up visit or consultation.
- Measuring any relevant physiological or functional criteria (e.g. peak flow rate, pulse, or the amount of fluid spilt on elevating cup to lip).
- Comparing measurements with the baseline measurement.
- Asking for the views of the old person.
- Asking the opinion of carers.
- Deciding whether further action is needed.

Helping trainees acquire these skills   Having helped the trainee develop a problem-orientated approach, it is also necessary to help him or her to develop a systematic approach to follow-up. Note that hospital practice does not give junior doctors the opportunity to think about planning treatment and follow-up over the course of a year or an even longer period of time.

Recording the impact of treatment   The sheet used for recording problems and objectives can also be used for recording the impact of treatment by having a column for information collected at follow-up. If a problem is solved in follow-up, then that particular row on the table can be closed. If the problem is not solved but requires further interventions then either additional follow-ups can be planned, or, if some progress has been made, a new sheet can be started with a new problem.

14 Adaptations to the home: the contribution of the occupational therapist

Introduction

The home environment of an older person can be potentially dangerous, the hazards ranging from those that make it more likely they will slip and fall, to others that may play a part in increasing confusion and disorientation. Careful assessment and organization of the environment will allow the person living in it to lead as independent a life in the community as possible, for as long as possible.

Some problems and hazards are relatively easily solved, while others will require more expert advice. The solution to many problems is often one of common sense, and although some advice in respect of particular problems will be offered in this chapter, it is important to realize that every situation is unique. Environmental problems may also be compounded by the differing standards and expectations of different individuals. An experienced occupational therapist will usually be able to help by offering advice for the more complex situations.

The most important specific problems are presented below, with suggestions that are often found helpful set out in the form of a check-list, which could be given to District Nurses and Health Visitors as a preventive measure, as well as being used to help solve problems that have already arisen.

Mobility

General

- Avoid trailing flexes
- Remove loose rugs and carpets, or tape them down (suitable double-sided sticky tape is available)
- Avoid shiny floors
- Rails by steps
- Trolley for transporting items from room to room
- Sitting at sink instead of standing for kitchen activities
- Pendant or wrist alarm system for use after a fall
- A basket or something similar can be fixed to a zimmer frame, so that both hands are free to use the frame whilst transporting objects.
- Fire guards

Unsteadiness on stairs

- Additional stair rails
- Stair lift (this is expensive and often difficult to obtain from social services)
- Bring bed downstairs
- Do not forget the need for suitable toilet facilities or commode
- Improve carpeting and lighting on existing stairway
- Convert steep steps into a greater number of smaller steps if possible.

Unsteadiness outdoors

- Wheelchair for long distance (need to make sure there is an able attendant)
- Ramp access (for wheelchair users only). Ramps are more difficult for pedestrians, especially in bad weather.

Problems with transferring

Bed

- Raise or lower bed height, as appropriate
- Board between mattress and bed to make mattress firmer
- Monkey poles and 'rope ladders' to help a person sit up in bed

Chair

- Raise chair height
- Ejector seats/chairs to ease standing

Toilet

- Rails around the toilet
- High seat

Bath

- Bath aids, especially grab rails and non-slip mats both inside and outside the bath
- Ensure someone is around when bathing.

Bending difficulties

- Raise electric plugs
- Refer to Gas Board to raise taps and knobs on gas fires
- Use 'helping hand' to pick up items from the floor
- Long-handled aids, e.g. shoehorn, milk-bottle holder

Sensory loss

Visual

- Bright-coloured sticky labels to show up items, e.g. cooker knobs
- Large telephone numbers
- Improve lighting
- Paint edge of steps if possible
- There are a variety of other aids available from RNIB (the Royal National Institute for the Blind)

Hearing

- Flashing door bell
- Amplifier for telephone

Tactile

- Educate about loss of sensation.

Lack of dexterity

There are a number of aids available, e.g.

- Tap-turners
- Jar-openers
- Dycem mat
- Dressing sticks
- Kettle-tippers.

Poor memory and disorientation

- Reminding signs, e.g. to turn cooker off
- Disconnect cooker if continually unsafe and replace with mobile meals and snacks
- Avoid trying to establish new routine or introducing new labour-saving environments because it may be impossible for the patient to learn to use them
- Put a list of items on the front of drawers and cupboards
- Ensure all clocks and calendars are correct.

Additional points

The 'helping hand' aid is very useful in many instances, but some people do not have the manual dexterity to make the most use of it. As well as picking things up that are beyond easy reach, a shorter aid of this nature can help with dressing the lower part of the body. Aids to help a person put on their socks and stockings are also valuable, but not everyone for whom they may seem suitable will be able to use one.

Where it has proved difficult to alter the height of switches, etc., a piece of dowel with a rubber thimble on the end can be used to switch on and off electrical points, and if a hook is placed on the other end, this can be used to help with cord-pull switches, etc., such as are found in most modern bathrooms. This simple tool is also adaptable for helping with many other problems.

Wandering can also be a problem, if only because sometimes preventing wandering can result in the person concerned becoming more disturbed, and possible aggressive. Apart from obvious measures such as making sure that external doors are locked, it is often a good idea to put potentially hazardous objects in one room, locking the door to this as well. Most confused wanderers will merely move to another door if they find they cannot open the one in front of them.

If wandering at night is a problem, thick black curtains may prevent light from entering the bedroom and being misinterpreted as an indication that it is time to get up. A night-light on the landing is also helpful, and may prevent a confused wanderer from tripping, or falling down the stairs.

Should it prove impossible to divert a confused person's attention from an external door, placing a curtain in front of it may well adequately disguise its presence, and divert attention elsewhere.

Where aids and changes to the home are concerned, it is important to remember that one can only advise and not enforce changes or new routines. Responsibility for safety falls largely on the patient and his or her relatives, and they can take or refuse the advice of professional people, as they feel appropriate, except in those very rare circumstances when they may be made the subject of a compulsory order.

Conclusion

A simple check-list of the sort presented above can go a long way to help make an elderly person more secure in the home environment. It is very important however not to forget that if this proves inadequate, as it often will do, further advice should be sought from an occupational therapist.

Appendix

As an example of occupational therapists in action, there now follows an anonymized, verbatim report from an occupational therapist on one of our patients, carried out at the request of the GP acting before the patient was discharged following hip surgery after being blown over in her garden.

DoB: ...

GP: ...

Consultant: ...

Diagnosis: Left dynamic hip screw

Date of visit: ...

Reason for visit: To assess Miss T's ability to manage at home alone.

Those present: Miss T—patient
Ms L. J.—occupational therapist
Ms J. B.—occupational therapy student
Ms A. B.—social worker
Dr J. M. L.—general practitioner.

Home situation   Miss T lives alone in her own cottage. Prior to her admission she had a cat, which was being looked after by a neighbour, Mrs B, who has now found it too much and has given it away. Mrs B does give some support. Storm damage to the conservatory.

Access: No garden path. Clear, but muddy access over uneven grass to front door. Rest of the garden is overgrown, especially at the back. Not safe managing the two steps to the front door, which then opens over the lounge door. Does not use the back door.

Mobility: Walks independently on the level with two sticks. Stairs: as ascent—open plan to left, and rope to support on right (half way up only) 180° turn with narrowing of stairs. Ascend further six stairs with support on right. With one stick needed minimal verbal supervision and minimal physical help to steady on ascending and descending. At this time was not independent or safe. Did not see dead rat which happened to be at the foot of the stairs.

Activities of daily living: Washing: independent on ward.
Dressing: still needs help to put pants, socks, and slippers on.
Toileting: manages independently.

Lounge: Chair: independent in/out.
Unable to plug fan heater into low socket—appeared to be eyesight problems—does not wear glasses. Room was very cluttered and dirty with old newspapers and magazines limiting clear walking space.

Kitchen: Chair: independent in/out using kitchen table as support. Walked independently using a trolley although limited space. Very cluttered and dirty—poor hygiene. Managed to make a cup of tea independently and safely, but had difficulty lighting gas. (Matches damp and igniter not working.) May have problems lighting oven.

Bathroom: Downstairs—no toilet upstairs.
Toilet: independent on/off.
Bath not assessed.

Bedroom: Bed: independent on/off.
Has electric fire upstairs—kept on landing, plugged into spare room (adjacent) and pulled through to bedroom. Room was very untidy with clean and dirty clothes strewn everywhere.

Domestic activities: Shopping: neighbour gives lift to shops.
Cleaning ⎤ Says she managed these herself
Cooking ⎦ prior to admission.

Recommendations:
1 Have industrial cleaners employed to clean and tidy Miss T's cottage *prior* to her return home.
2 Request social services to provide the following:
Two grab rails at the front door.
Bath equipment.
3 Ophthalmic referral.
4 Extra stick to be kept at the top of stairs.
5 Further practice to increase independence in the following:
  • Dressing practice
  • Bath pratice
  • Kitchen work
  • Stairs
  • Plugging in and unplugging equipment safely.
6 Referral to Home Care Services.

Conclusion: Miss T managed transfers safely, although the limited floor space within the cottage was hazardous to her mobility. The cottage was unkempt, dirty, and very cluttered, and, as Miss T agreed, needed to be sorted out. When this has occurred she will require a further home visit prior to discharge. With the above recommendation, and any others from the second visit, Miss T should be able to manage at home alone.

It is easy to skim over these reports from occupational therapists when they are read after a busy surgery—without really appreciating their value. To do this, one must be present at the home visit oneself. Hidden behind this occupational therapist's report are a number of crucial areas for discussion and illumination. For example, at the beginning of the home visit, Miss T apparently did not seem aware of the total chaos of her dwelling, or its unhygienic state. The occupational therapist could easily have confronted her with the evidence of her own eyes—but wisely she did not. Instead she spent time building up a good relationship with Miss T. Revealingly, towards the end of the visit, Miss T began to apologize for the state of her house—and it was then that the offer for help was accepted. It is easy to object that we are too busy to take time to go on these lengthy visits, but it is worth pointing out the benefits of these visits both to the patient, and to the professionals involved. In these visits we have, as it were, a microcosm of the National Health Service in action, providing a level of care that cannot be bettered anywhere: four professionals gathered together with the patient, in her own home, finding out in deail about an elderly person's way of life, and offering support and practical help from their own linked perspectives. We should not underestimate the humanizing effects of these meetings of minds. The patient, who up until now has been a recluse, spontaneously came out of herself, and the staff demonstrated a reawakening of professional ideals and motivation in themselves.

At the time of writing, we do not yet know the outcome of Miss T's discharge. Perhaps she will trip over as soon as she arrives home, and fracture the other hip—and the whole exercise will have been wasted; but for all we know Miss T's home visit may have been the start of her abandoning her reclusive life-style, and her re-emergence into the community. It is also true to say that at the time of writing we do not know whether there will be much space left for this sort of intensive and inspiring intervention in the post-reform NHS, where the computer will see you now, please; and if you are old, demented, or needing many expensive drugs, you will not be an attractive proposition to the buyers, purveyors, and human auctioneers in our new health market. It is our surmise that if we redouble our vigilance and make our priorities widely known the best of our health service may yet be retained.

Part IV   Appendices

Appendix 1. Useful addresses

Abbeyfield Society, 29 Hereford Road, Shrewsbury SY3 7QX, tel: 0743 52078/61884

Age Concern, (England), Bernard Sunnley House, 60 Pitcairne Road, Mitcham, Surrey CR4 3LL, tel: 081 640 5431

Age Concern (Ireland), 6 Lower Crescent, Belfast BT7 1NR, tel: 0232 245729

Age Concern (Scotland), 33 Castle Street, Edinburgh EH2 3DM, tel: 031 556 5000

Age Concern (Wales), 1 Park Grove, Cadiff, CF1 3BJ, tel: 0222 371821

Alzheimer's Disease Society, Head Office, 158/160 Balham High Road, London SW12 9BN: 081 675 6557

Regional Offices:

LONDON—St Botolph without Aldersgate, Aldersgate Street, London EC1A 4EV, tel: 071 726 8617

SOUTH-WEST—Hettling House, 2 Hettling Court, Bath BA1 1SH, tel: 0225 69402/69460

MIDLANDS—70/76 Alcester Road South, Kings Heath, Birmingham B14 7PT, tel: 021 444 5424

NORTH—The Poplars, Holgate, St Barnabas Road, Middlesborough, Cleveland TS5 6BZ, tel: 0642 820921/2

EASTERN COUNTIES—185 Great North Road, Eaton Socon, St Neots, Cambs PE19 3EE, tel: 0480 406567

WESSEX—Room 6, Nightingale Clnic, Wilton Road, Salisbury, tel: 0722 26236

Anchor Housing Association, Oxonford House, 13/15 Magdalen Street, Oxford, OX1 3BP, tel: 0865 722261

Apollo Baths (with built-in, hydraulically operated seat-lift) Apollo House, 34 Church Road, Romsey, Hants, SO51 8ZT, Tel: 0794 523455

Arthritis Care, 6 Grovesnor Crescent, London SW1X 7ER, tel: 071 235 0902

Crossroad Care Attendant Scheme Trust, 10 Regents Place, Rugby, Warwickshire CV21 29N, tel: 0788 73653

The British Diabetic Association, 10 Queen Anne Street, London W1N 0BD, tel: 071 323 1531

The British Heart Foundation, 102 Gloucester Place, London W1H 4DH, tel: 071 935 0185

The British Red Cross Society, 9 Grosvenor Crescent, London SW1X 7EJ, tel: 071 235 5454

The British Talking Book Service for the Blind, Mount Pleasant, Wembley, Middx, HA2 1RR, tel: 081 903 6666

The Chest, Heart and Stroke Association, Tavistock House North, Tavistock Square, London WC1H 9JE, tel: 071 387 3012

Court of Protection, Chief Clerk to the Court of Protection 25 Store Street, London WC1E 7BT, tel: 071 636 6877

Cruse, Cruse House, 126 Sheen Road, Richmond, Surrey, TW9 1UR, tel: 081 940 4818/9047

Disabled Living Foundation, 380/384 Harrow Road, London W9 1HU, tel: 071 289 6111

The Disablement Income Group, Abbey House, 28 Commercial Street, London E1 6LR, tel: 071 247 2128/6877

Friends of the Elderly and Gentlefolks Help, 42 Ebury Street, London SW1W 0L2, tel: 071 730 8236

Help the Aged, St James Walk, London EC1R 0BE, tel: 071 253 0253

Methodist Homes for the Aged, Epworth House, 25 City Road, London EC1Y 1DR, tel: 081 368 1431

National Council for Carers and their Dependents, 29 Chilworth Mews, London W2 3RG, tel: 071 262 1451/2

The Parkinson's Disease Society, 36 Portland Place, London W1N 3DG, tel: 071 323 1174

The Registered Nursing Homes Association, 7a Station Road, London N3 2SB

The Royal National Institute for the Blind, 224 Great Portland Street, London W1N 6AA, tel: 071 388 1266

The Royal National Institute for the Deaf, 105 Gower Street, London WC1E 6AH, tel: 071 387 8033

Talking Newspapers U.K., 68A High Street, Heathfield, East Sussex, TN21 8JB, tel: 04352 6102

Women's Royal Voluntary Service, 234/244 Stockwell Road, London SW9 9SP, tel: 071 733 3388

Appendix 2.   The coroner

To a certain extent coroners themselves determine what information they require after a death has occurred, if any is necessary at all. The coroner's officer, usually a police officer especially seconded to work with the coroner, is always pleased to inform doctors of the local coroner's views and statutory requirements. The coroner's officer is also usually very experienced and able to give unofficial as well as official advice about the best way of approaching a particular problem, and will always advise when there is any doubt about the need to refer a particular case. In general, however, if there is indeed any doubt it is better to refer the matter to the coroner. Referral is usually necessary if a death occurs without any obvious cause within 24 hours of admission to hospital, and this is so even when it is the local community or cottage hospital that is involved. Any suggestion of 'unnatural means' having contributed to a patient's demise also necessitates automatic referral to the coroner. Finally, any situation in which the issue of a death certificate presents difficulties, especially if there is a possibility of violence, should also automatically be discussed with the coroner.

The coroner and coroner's officer are usually extremely helpful, making it their responsibility to look after the proper interests of the medical profession, as well as members of the general public. An inquest rarely results following the referral of a death to the coroner unless the circumstances are exceptional, although a post-mortem will often be necessary.

In Scotland, these duties are performed by the Procurator Fiscal.

Appendix 3. Compulsory institutionalization

Compulsory hospitalization of psychiatrically ill patients

Introduction

The 1983 Mental Health Act has superseded its 1959 predecessor and has particularly tried to safeguard further the interests and rights of patients subject to treatment for psychiatric problems. The first section is mainly concerned with definition of the terms in the remainder of the Act. Other relevant sections are summarized below.

Section II

Admission for assessment for a maximum of 28 days. This allows compulsory admission for both assessment of mental condition and also treatment. It has to be initiated by the nearest relative or an approved social worker, and two doctors must support the recommendations. One of the medical practitioners has to be approved under the Act for this purpose. Medical recommendations have to confirm that the patient's mental disorder requires detention for assessment and also that detention is necessary in the interest of the patient's own health or safety, or for the protection of others. Discharge is via the Mental Health Review tribunal, the nearest relative, the hospital managers, or the responsible medical officer. The latter can in certain circumstances prevent the nearest relative arranging the discharge.

Section III

Admission for treatment for a maximum of 6 months. Again the nearest relative or an approved social worker can make the application, which must be supported by a medical recommendation from two doctors, one of whom is approved under the Act. The patient has to be suffering from mental illness, mental impairment, or psychopathic disorder requiring treatment in hospital. For mental impairment or a psychopathic disorder there must be the likelihood that treatment will alleviate or prevent deterioration and be necessary for the health and safety of the patient or the protection of other people. This section can be extended. The patient has a right to appeal within six months of admission and also during any period of extension.

Section IV

Admission for assessment in cases of emergency—up to 72 hours. The nearest relative or an approved social worker and one doctor, who preferably will be acquainted with the patient, can make the application. The grounds for admission are the same as in section II except that the degree of urgency is sufficient that invoking section II would result in undesirable delay.

Section V (ii)

Application in respect of a patient already in hospital, for a maximum of 72 hours. This section allows any patient already receiving treatment in hospital to be held for a period of up to 72 hours. The doctor in charge of the case, or his nominated deputy, may make the application on the grounds that the patient is dangerous to himself or others. Detention can only be continued after 72 hours if section II or section III are then invoked.

Section 58

Treatment requiring consent or a second opinion. This is most usually required when ECT is being considered, although in future the Secretary of State may specify other forms of treatment that may fall within this section. Before the administration of treatment listed in this section to a detained patient:

(a) the responsible medical officer or an independent doctor must certify in writing that the patient is capable of understanding the nature of the treatment, its purpose and likely effects, and has consented. The patient must clearly also have consented.

(b) OR an independent doctor must specify in writing that although the patient is not capable of understanding the nature, purpose, and likely effects of the treatment, or has not consented to it, it should nevertheless be given as it may alleviate or prevent deterioration of the condition.

It is very important that the independent doctor consults two other people who have been professionally involved with the patient's medical treatment and takes into account their knowledge and opinion before giving his own clinical decision. Of these two other people, one must be a nurse and the other must be neither a nurse nor a doctor.

Appendix 4. Compulsory removal of the physically ill and disabled

The 1951 amendment of Section 47 of the National Assistance Act 1948 is usually involved.

Two medical practitioners, one a community physician approved for this purpose by the appropriate Health Authority and the other usually, but not always, the patient's own GP certify that it is in the interest of the patient to be removed without delay because he is:

(a) Suffering from grave chronic disease, or being aged, infirm or physically incapacitated, is living in insanitary conditions and

(b) Is unable to devote to himself and is not receiving from other persons, proper care and attention.

It can sometimes be invoked because a patient is a danger to others. A Magistrate or Justice of the Peace must be involved before the Order can be made. The Order allows detention for up to 3 weeks in a suitable place, e.g. hospital.

Section 47 itself allows the approved community physician to arrange compulsory detention in a suitable institution for up to three months, but in these circumstances seven clear days notice have to be given to the person concerned.

In an emergency the general practitioner should be able to contact an approved medical practitioner, as each Health Authority usually has a rota. They are usually community physicians.

Appendix 5. Court of Protection and Power of Attorney

The Court of Protection protects and controls the administration of affairs and property of a person with a mental disorder which makes him incapable of managing his own affairs. This is particularly relevant to the elderly, but is probably only worth using if significant assets are involved. An Official Receiver will be appointed by the Court after a solicitor has submitted an 'originating application', but the Court will also consider personal applications. The 'originating application' is usually initiated by a near relative, with the solicitor's help, and it is usual for the relative who will be appointed as the 'Receiver' to be the initiator of the application. The doctor has to prepare and sign an affidavit about the patient's mental state and other matters, and will eventually have to serve upon the patient a notice informing him that his affairs will be considered by the Court on a particular date. The patient has seven days to make an objection, either against the need for an Order to be made or against the proposed 'Receiver'. The patient can give his own view of how his property should be managed and who he feels would be the most appropriate 'Receiver'.

A Power of Attorney is usually arranged when a person of sound mind voluntarily and knowingly gives a second person legal responsibility for the management of his financial affairs, either in a general sense or for a particular purpose. The Deed is drawn up by a solicitor, but this arrangement ceases to be valid when the person on whose behalf the Power of Attorney has been drawn up becomes of unsound mind. This has caused many problems in the past, particularly in respect of dementia in the elderly, and the situation has now, thankfully, been eased by the possibility of being able to establish an 'Enduring Power of Attorney'. In this case a person can, when of sound mind, make legal arrangements for the second person to continue with the arrangement should the intellectual ability of the person delegating responsibility decline. A solicitor will be able to provide further advice about this when necessary.

Appendix 6. A table of normal values in the elderly

Serum/plasma	SI units
Albumin	33–50 g/l
Alkaline phosphatase	80–280 iu/l
Bilirubin	2–17 μmol/l
Calcium	2.15–2.6 mmol/l
Creatinine	52–160 μmol/l
ESR—men	0–20 mm in the first hour*
—women	0–30 mm in the first hour*
Glucose (random)	3.5–9.3 mmol/l
LDH	230–530 units/ml
Potassium	3.5–4.8 mmol/l
AST (aspartate transaminase)	5–40 units/ml
Sodium	133–145 mmol/l
Total T4	58–128 nom/l
Total T3	1.0–3.0 nmol/l
TSH	0.35–6 mu/l
Urea	4–10 mmol/l

* The ESR increases with age. The above is a rough guide. A more reliable way to calculate the upper limit of normal (in men) is their age in years ÷ 2. In women the formula is: (age in years + 10) ÷ 2 (Miller 1983).

Appendix 7. The mini-mental-state examination

If dementia is suspected test memory and other intellectual abilities formally. The mini-mental-state examination* is one of many similar tests; it has been more fully studied than most.

- **What day of the week is it?**
- **What is the date today? Day; Month; Year** [One point each.]
- **What is the season?** [Allow flexibility when testing in March (i.e. Winter or Spring), June, September, December.]
- **Can you tell me where we are now? What country are we in?**
- **What is the name of this town?**
- **What are two main streets nearby?**
- **What floor of the building are we on?**
- **What is the name of this place?** (or what is this address?)
- Read the following, then proffer the paper: **'I am going to give you a piece of paper. When I do, take the paper in your right hand. Fold the paper in half with both hands and put the paper down on your lap.'** [Give one point for each of the three actions.]
- **Show a pencil and ask what it is called.**
- **Show a wristwatch and ask what it is called.**
- Say (once only): **'I am going to say something and I would like you to repeat it after me: No ifs, ands, or buts.'** [Speak clearly.]
- Say: **'Please read what is written here and do what it says.'** [Show card with: CLOSE YOUR EYES written on it.] Score only if action is carried out correctly. If respondent reads instruction but fails to carry out action, say: 'Now do what it says'.

Close your eyes.

- Say: **'Write a complete sentence on this sheet of paper.'** Spelling and grammar are not important. The sentence must have a verb, real or implied, and must make sense. 'Help!', 'Go away' are acceptable.

* M. Folstein (1975) *J. Psychiatric Research* **12,** 189–98

- Say: **'Here is a drawing. Please copy the drawing.'** [See drawing below.] Mark as correct if the two figures intersect to form a four-sided figure and if all angles are preserved.

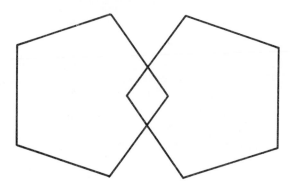

- Say: **'I am going to name three objects. After I have finished saying all three I want you to repeat them. Remember what they are because I am going to ask you name them again in a few minutes.'** [Name three objects taking 1 second to say each, e.g. APPLE; TABLE; PENNY.] Score first try (one point each object) and repeat until all are learned.
- Say: **'Now I would like you to take 7 away from 100. Now take 7 away from the number you get. Now keep subtracting until I tell you to stop.'** Score 1 point each time the difference is 7 even if a previous answer was incorrect. Continue until 5 subtractions (e.g. 93, 86, 79, 72, 65).
- Say: **'What were the three objects I asked you to repeat a little while ago?'** [One point each object.]

Interpreting the score

The maximum is 30. Score 28–30 does not support the diagnosis of dementia. Score 25–27 is borderline. Score <25 suggests dementia but consider also *acute confusional state* and *depression*.

References

Abrams, M. (1978) *Beyond three score and ten*. Age Concern, London.

Age Concern (1988) *The living will. Consent to treatment at the end of life*. Edward Arnold, London.

Anand, J. K., Pryor G. A., and Morgon R. T. T. (1989) Hospital at home. *Health Trends* **21**, 46–8.

Beauchamp T. C. and Childrers J. F. (1983) *Principles of Biomedical Ethics*. OUP, New York.

British Medical Association *Euthanasia* 1988 (Report of the working party to review the BMA's guidance on euthanasia)

Brockington C. F. and Lampert S. M. (1966) *The social needs of the over 80s*. Manchester University Press.

Bass C. (1989) *Brit. Med. J.* **ii**, 345.

Bullock N. (1985) *Brit. Med. J.* **291**, 1522.

Cassidy S. and Henry J. (1987) *Brit. Med. J.* **295**, 1021–4.

Coleman P. (1989) The value of screening the elderly. *Family Practitioner Service* **16:9** (October) 424.

Drug Ther. Bul. **27** (10) 37–9 (1989) Treating depression in the elderly.

Gillon R. (1988) Euthanasia, withholding life-prolonging treatment, and moral differences between killing and letting die. *Journal of Medical Ethics* **14**, 115–7.

Gloag D. (1990) Fit for living. *Brit. Med. J.* **300**, 351.

Glorig A. (1957) *Wisconsin State Fair hearing survey*. Rochester, Minnesota: American Academy of Ophthalmology and Otolaryngology.

Griffin J. P. and Chew R. (1990) Trends in usage of prescription medicines by the elderly and very elderly between 1977 and 1988. The Association of the British Pharmaceutical Industry, 12 Whitehall, London SW1A 2DY.

Harris C. (1988) Abuse of the elderly. *Brit.Med J.* **297**, 813–4.

Harris A. T. (1988) Appointment systems: evaluation of a flexible system offering patients a limited choice. *Brit. Med. J.* **296**, 685–6.

Hickish G. (1989) Hearing problems of the elderly. *Brit.Med. J.* **299**, 1415–6.

Hunt, A. (1978) *The elderly at home*. HMSO, London.

Illich I. (1976) *Limits to medicine*. Boyars.

Kalache A. (1988) *Promoting health among elderly people*. (Working Party Statement) King's Fund Institute, London.

Kellett, J. M. (1989) Sex and the elderly. *Brit. Med. J.* **299**, 934.

Langer R. D., Ganiats T. G., and Barrett-Connor, E. (1989) Paradoxical survival of elderly men with high blood pressure. *Brit. Med. J.* **298**, 1356–7.

Lawton F. G. and Hacker N. F. (1989) Sex and the elderly. *Brit. Med. J.* **299**, 1279.

Longmore J. M. (1986) *An Atlas of Bedside Microscopy*. Royal College of General Practitioners Occasional Paper number 32.

Lowry S. (1989) Temperature and humidity. *Brit. Med. J.* **299**, 1326–8.

Miller A. (1983) *Brit Med. J.* **i**, 266.

Morgan, M. J. (1989) Looking after a patient with Alzheimer's disease. *Brit. Med. J.* **299**, 1606–7.

Parkinson's Study Group (1989) Effect of deprenyl on the progression of disability in early Parkinson's disease. *New Eng. J. Med.* **321**, 1364–71.

Rabbitt P. (1988) Social psychology, neurosciences and cognitive psychology need each other; (and gerontology needs all three of them) *The Psychologist: Bulletin of the British Psychological Society* **12**, 500–6.

Rachel J. (1975) Active and passive euthanasia *New Eng. J. Med.* **292**, 78–80.

Regnard C. (1986) *A Guide to Symptom Relief in Advanced Cancer*, distributed by Haigh & Hochland—tel 061 273 4156 (ISBN 1 869888 00 6)

Rogstad K. E. and Bignell C. J.(1989) Sex and the elderly *Brit. Med. J.* **299**, 1279.

Rowntree B. S. (1947) Report of the survey committee on the problems of aging and the care of old people. Nuffield Foundation.

Sheldon J. H. (1948) *The social medicine of old age*. Oxford.

Smedira N. G., Evans B. H., Gravis L. S., Cohen N. H. *et al*. (1990) Withholding and withdrawing life support from the critically ill. *New Eng. J. Med.* **322**. 309–15.

Salthouse, A. (1985) *A theory of cognitive ageing*, Berlin, Springer.

Stoate, H. G. (1989) Can health screening damage your health? *Journal of the Royal College of General Practitioners* **39**, 193–5.

Stringfellow (1989) *Monitor* 2 (41) 15.

Tinetti M. E. and Speechley M. (1989) Prevention of falls among the elderly. *New Eng. J. Med.* **320**, 1055–9.

Wallston, K. A. *et al*. (1988) Comparing the quality of death for hospice and non-hospice cancer patients. *Med. Care* **26** (2), 177–82.

Whitehead M. (1987) *The health divide*. Health Education Council.

Williamson J., Stoke I. H., Gray S., Fisher M., Smith A., McGhee A., and Stephenson E. (1964) Old people at home, their unreported needs. *Lancet* **i**, 1117–20.

Wood P. H. N. (1980) The language of disablement. *International Rehabilitation Medicine* **2**, 86–92.

Index

statistics, population 3, 4–15
sterile pyuria 123, 129
steroids 59, 80, 89, 90, 129
stockings, elastic 116
street registers 174
streptomycin 130
stress incontinence 100
stress on carers 55
strokes 52, 62–6, 93–4
subacute bacterial endocarditis 138
subdural haematoma 52, 63, 126
sulphonylureas 72, 150
surgery
  arthritis 59, 60
  pressure sores 121–2
sympathy 157–8
syptoms
  control for terminal care 162–4
  incidence 9

tamponade, cardiac 53
team practices 188
temperatures, room 93
temporal arteritis 80–1
temporal lobe function 66
terminal care 152–65
  drugs 163–4
terodiline 101
tertiary prevention 170–9
tetanus vaccination 170
tetracyclines 149
thiazides 148
thrombolytic therapy 35
thyroid disorders 126–8
thyrotoxicosis 128, 138
thyrotrophin-releasing hormone test 127, 128
thyroxine therapy 127–8
time for listening 154, 156
tinnitus 131
toe-nails, cutting 94
tolbutamide 72
training, GP 201–2, 204–5
tranquillizers 146–8
tricyclic antidepressants 69, 100, 163, 164
triiodothyronine levels 127–8
trust 152–4
tuberculin tests 129–30
tuberculosis 129–30, 138
Tubigrip 116
24-hour urine collections 90
twilight district nurses 50, 161

ulcers
  leg 109–11
  peptic 137
ultraviolet light therapy 122
uninhibited neurogenic bladder 101
urea levels (blood) 122
urgency of micturition 98
uric acid levels 60
uricosuric drugs 60
urinary tract infection 124
urine
  bile pigments 108–9
  collections (24-hour) 90
  incontinence 98–105
  osmolality 91
urobilinogen 109

vaccination 170
vaginitis, senile 100
value of old people 35–6
varicose ulcers 109
vascular disease, ulcers 110
vasodilators 149
venodilators 62
venous obstruction 115
vertigo 75, 130–1
visual impairment 132–6
  adaptation of home for 211
vitamin B_{12} deficiency 56–7
vitamin D
  deficiency 88
  therapy 117
voluntary organizations 184
volunteer sitters 50
vomiting 90, 91

waiting-lists for beds 189–92
walking frames 96
wandering 212
water retention 91
weakness, generalized 93
wealth of old people 3
weight loss 136–9
wills, living 30–5
Woodside 9-item screening letter 172

X-rays
  osteomalacia 117
  tuberculosis 129

Zimmer frames 96